Obesity

Obesity

Global Impact and Epidemiology

Edited by

Raman Mehrzad, M.D., M.H.L., M.B.A.
Physician, Plastic and Reconstructive Surgery, Rhode Island Hospital,
Brown University, Providence, RI, United States

ELSEVIER

Elsevier
Radarweg 29, PO Box 211, 1000 AE Amsterdam, Netherlands
The Boulevard, Langford Lane, Kidlington, Oxford OX5 1GB, United Kingdom
50 Hampshire Street, 5th Floor, Cambridge, MA 02139, United States

Library of Congress Cataloging-in-Publication Data
A catalog record for this book is available from the Library of Congress

British Library Cataloguing-in-Publication Data
A catalogue record for this book is available from the British Library

ISBN: 978-0-12-818839-2

For information on all Elsevier publications
visit our website at https://www.elsevier.com/books-and-journals

Publisher: Stacy Masucci
Acquisitions Editor: Ana Claudia A. Garcia
Editorial Project Manager: Pat Gonzalez
Production Project Manager: Omer Mukthar
Cover Designer: Matthew Limbert

Typeset by SPi Global, India

Contents

Contributors

Numbers in parenthesis indicate the pages on which the authors' contributions begin.

Jacqueline Chu, B.A. (7, 85), The Ohio State University College of Medicine, Columbus, OH, United States

Lindsey G. Kahan, B.S. (117, 165), Department of Plastic and Reconstructive Surgery, Rhode Island Hospital, The Warren Alpert Medical School of Brown University, Providence, RI, United States

David Kim, M.D. (183, 191), Department of Surgery, Rhode Island Hospital, Alpert Medical School of Brown University, Providence, RI, United States

Elizabeth Kiwanuka, M.D., Ph.D. (73, 99, 109), Department of Plastic Surgery, Rhode Island Hospital, Providence, RI, United States

Raman Mehrzad, M.D., M.H.L., M.B.A. (1, 7, 19, 43, 55, 85, 117, 165), Department of Plastic and Reconstructive Surgery, Rhode Island Hospital, The Warren Alpert Medical School of Brown University, Providence, RI, United States

Zohra Salehi, M.D., Pharm.D. (141, 155), Hospital Medicine, Hartford HealthCare, Hartford, CT, United States

Ollin Venegas, B.A. (19), Department of Plastic and Reconstructive Surgery, Rhode Island Hospital, The Warren Alpert Medical School of Brown University, Providence, RI, United States

Preface

The World Health Organization has declared obesity a global epidemic. Its prevalence has more than doubled since 1980, causing a myriad of health problems for children and adults. Today, more than one-third of the world's population is classified as obese or overweight. If this trend continues, researchers estimate that by the year 2030, this number will reach more than 50%. Although recognized clinically as an important condition that increases the risk of multiple diseases and is a major contributor to morbidity and mortality, it is only in recent years that obesity has been identified as a population-wide problem that requires preventive action. Due to its complex and multifactorial nature, however, prevention and slowing the incidences have been challenging.

In order to know where we can go, we need to know where we are in this major epidemic. Therefore, epidemiological studies in obesity are of utmost importance because they identify risk factors that may represent critical control points for this global problem. Moreover, obesity is an evolving field with continuous research being pursued by numerous medical specialties and scientists around the world. Each year, multiple new studies and evidence-based guidelines are being published on this topic. Therefore, this book offers the latest science in the field of obesity epidemiology that analyzes the distribution (who, when, and where), patterns, and determinants of obesity. This book will depict everything from analytic epidemiology designs in obesity research to prevalence and trends in obesity in the United States and affluent countries to environmental and cultural factors related to the obesity epidemic to obesity's consequences and conditions in defined populations around the globe.

The target audience for this book includes the majority of folks in the medical field, as obesity is an area related to almost every field in medicine. More specifically, healthcare professionals in the fields of general surgery, plastic surgery, internal medicine, endocrinology, obesity medicine, cardiology, and gastroenterology as well as Ph.D. students and scientists focusing on metabolism obesity research will benefit from this book immensely. Medical students, nursing students, nurse practitioners, physician assistants, medical residents, and fellows are also students that would find value in this book.

Raman Mehrzad, M.D., M.H.L., M.B.A.

Chapter 1

Definition and introduction to epidemiology of obesity

Raman Mehrzad, M.D., M.H.L., M.B.A.
Department of Plastic and Reconstructive Surgery, Rhode Island Hospital, The Warren Alpert Medical School of Brown University, Providence, RI, United States

Overview and definition of obesity

Obesity is a global, complex, multifactorial, and generally preventable disease [1]. The global prevalence of obesity has doubled in the past 40 years regardless of sex, age, ethnicity, or socioeconomic status. Today, more than one-third of the world's population is classified as obese or overweight [2]. If this trend continues, researchers estimate that by 2030, this number will surpass 50% [3].

Obesity is typically defined as excess body weight for height. Today, due to its simplicity and low cost, body mass index (BMI), defined as the weight in kilograms divided by the height in meters squared (kg/m^2), is the most common measure of obesity. The National Institutes of health (NIH) and the World Health Organization (WHO) define overweight as having a BMI between 25.0 and 29.9 kg/m^2, and obesity as having a BMI $>30.0\,kg/m^2$ [4, 5].

For children, the criteria for overweight are based on the 2000 US Centers for Disease Control and Prevention (CDC) BMI-for-age growth charts in the United States. Here, at or above the age-specific 95% BMI percentile is defined as overweight. Those at risk for overweight are defined as having a BMI between the 85th to 95th percentiles of the BMI-for-age growth chart [6].

Recently, there has been more evidence suggesting that abdominal fat rather than total body fat is an independent risk factor of cancer-related and cardiovascular outcomes. It has been suggested that the visceral and metabolically active fat surrounding the organs causes metabolic dysregulation, which in turn predisposes to disease. This is also known as the metabolic syndrome, which per international guidelines is a collection of dysmetabolic conditions that puts individuals at increased risk for cardiovascular disorders [7]. Nowadays, it is therefore common practice to measure the waist and hip circumference as well as the waist-to-hip ratio. It should be noted that the waist circumference that is defined to increase the risk for disease is different depending on race.

Obesity. https://doi.org/10.1016/B978-0-12-818839-2.00001-6

For instance, waist circumferences >94 cm in European men and >80 cm in European women are linked to higher cardiovascular risk, although in the Asian population, the cut-off is 90 vs. 80 cm for men and women, respectively [8].

Brief prevalence of obesity

Recent epidemiology studies have estimated that a total of 1.9 billion people worldwide were obese or overweight in 2015. This represents 39% of the world's population [3]. The prevalence is somewhat lower in women than men among ages 20–44; however, from 45 to 49, the trend reverses between the genders. Generally, obesity rates start to increase at 20 and peak between 50 and 65 with a slight decline subsequently. An increase of nearly 50% has been seen in the age-standardized prevalence in obesity over the past 3.5 decades, from 26.5% in 1980 to 39% in 2015, while the prevalence increased by 7% to 12.5% during the same time frame, accounting for an almost 80% increase [3]. Women had a greater rate of overweight and obesity than men in this period. The prevalence of obesity is largely uniform globally, although there are some variabilities between regions and countries [3].

Epidemiological studies

The purpose of epidemiological studies is to capture a baseline of where we stand on the issue of obesity as well as to identify the determinants and consequences to later find strategies for prevention and intervention. The epidemiology of obesity covers different research activities with the aim to study and monitor risk factors, consequences, and population trends, and to conduct studies on how to prevent and treat obesity [9].

Epidemiology studies in general are crucial to identify trends and patterns and later develop guidelines and recommendation for the population. Many of the current strategies have emerged from data of epidemiological studies [9]. For instance, the knowledge of the consequences of obesity has made us aware that this is a danger to health. Therefore, we now measure BMI and waist circumference, track the progress of weight gain and loss, etc. It has also resulted in emphasizing treatment options for patients that are at risk of obesity or are in the class of different stages of obesity. Therefore, continuous reports of these data are important to be able to refine our recommendations for patients and decrease mortality and morbidity. Moreover, studies on epidemiology encourage other research areas to actively analyze various molecular mechanisms, which further can identify targets for pharmaceutical approaches. A couple of examples of this are medications such as Orlistat (Xenical) and Lorcaserin (Belviq). These drugs target enzymes, receptors, and hormones that have been found to play a role in fat absorption and appetite [10, 11].

Multidisciplinary approach to obesity

Obesity is a multidisciplinary approach. Internists, cardiologists, endocrinologists, surgeons, dieticians, psychologists, and behavioral therapists are just a few that take care of patients with obesity. Although each provider may focus on specific areas, they are all needed in preventing and treating obesity. Likely, the cause of this is the complexity of the disease. Losing weight in a society where there are numerous temptations has been found to be difficult. Thus, providers from different specialties are needed to assist patients and optimize their results. In fact, studies show that a multidisciplinary approach is more effective for weight loss and maintenance [12–14].

Similarly, accurate study designs, valid measurements, experienced researchers, and collaboration between scientists and clinicians are important to make this research area optimal. Fig. 1 is a conceptualized flowchart that describes the different areas and interrelationships within epidemiological research.

Health consequences of obesity

Obesity has many serious health consequences. It adversely affects nearly all physiological functions in the body and increases the risks of cardiovascular diseases, hypertension, hyperlipidemia, chronic kidney disease, diabetes,

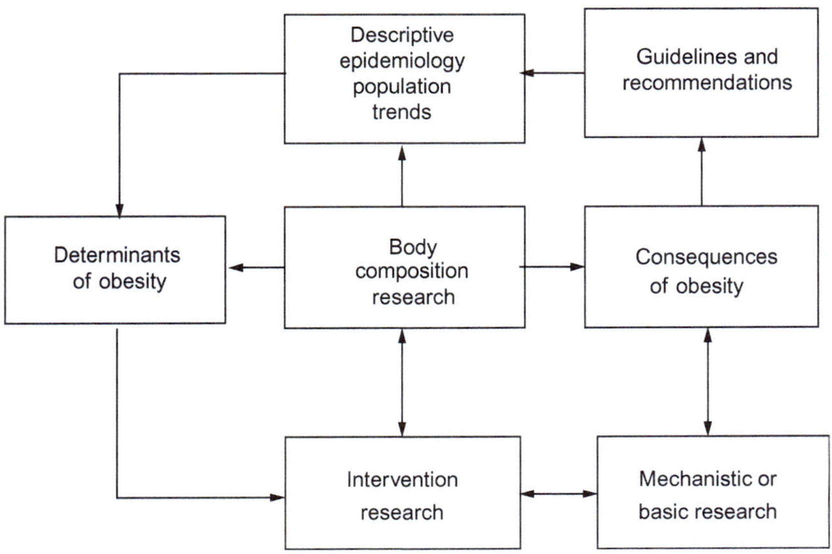

FIG. 1 Conceptual framework for the interrelationships among obesity epidemiology research domains. *(Adapted from Welk GJ. Introduction to physical activity research. In: Welk GJ, editor. Physical activity assessments for health-related research. Champaign, IL: Human Kinetics; 2000. p. 3–18.)*

cancers, musculoskeletal disorders, and poor mental health, just to name a few [15–19]. This area of research has grown significantly over the past few years, partly because obesity is an epidemic and partly because we now also have better quantitative methods in the field with the availability of body size or adiposity measurements in all epidemiological or clinical studies. Although these studies continue to improve our understanding of the disease and its healthcare consequences, there are still many questions that remain between the relationship of adiposity and how it brings different disease states as well as the impact of obesity on mortality [9]. To conduct studies that answer the above, careful considerations of epidemiological study design, analysis, and interpretation need to be made by scientists and clinicians.

Brief etiology of obesity

The etiology of obesity is molecularly simple to understand. A higher calorie intake than calorie expenditure results in a net positive calorie excess that in turn causes weight gain. Although this is simple mathematics, the actual regulation of body weight and fat is very complex and is a complicated interrelation of behavioral, genetic, endocrine, psychosocial, and environmental factors. Although we understand many of the causes of obesity, understanding these interrelations and other contributing factors remains to be elucidated. One of the issues with studies that determine the predictors of obesity is that they have many methodological problems such as reverse causation, confounding, and imprecise diet and physical exercise. In general, calorie intake and expenditure are many times subjective and not always easy to measure properly by patients or clinicians. Furthermore, obesity could at times bring certain behaviors and vice versa, and therefore reverse causation bias is a commonly encountered issue. These problems result in limitations when attempting to design study methods and make accurate conclusions.

Cost of obesity

The US health care costs of obesity are enormous. The cost of obesity is in the hundreds of billions in the United States per year as well as a significant portion of the gross domestic product in Europe when accounting for both direct and indirect costs. A more detailed report of the economic impact can be found in Chapter 5 [20, 21].

Goal of obesity research

The major objective to obesity research is to prevent it from happening and to treat those who are affected by it. Many studies on different dietary strategies and lifestyle modifications have been done at different levels: individual, community, school, and society. While we have many different tactics for the prevention and treatment of obesity, sufficient and sustainable interventions are yet to be found. This is true because regardless of the numerous strategies, the obesity trend is still growing, which proves that the problem is very complex [9].

References

[1] American Medical Association. AMA Adopts New Policies on Second Day of Voting at Annual Meeting. AMA; 2013. [Internet]. [cited 2014 Apr 7]. Available from: http://www.ama-assn.org/ama/pub/news/news/2013/2013-06-18-new-ama-policies-annual-meeting.page.

[2] IHME. Global burden of disease study 2015 (GBD 2015) obesity and overweight prevalence 1980–2015. Seattle, WA: Institute for Health Metrics and Evaluation (IHME); 2017.

[3] Chooi YC, Ding C, Magkos F. The epidemiology of obesity. Metabolism 2019 Mar;92:6–10. https://doi.org/10.1016/j.metabol.2018.09.005 [Epub 2018 Sep 22].

[4] World Health Organization. Obesity. WHO; 2008. Available at: http://www.who.int/topics/obesity/en. [Accessed 22 October 2009].

[5] Kumanyika SK, Obarzanek E, Stettler N, Bell R, Field AE, Fortmann SP, Franklin BA, Gillman MW, Lewis CE, Poston 2nd WC, Stevens J, Hong Y, American Heart Association Council on Epidemiology and Prevention, Interdisciplinary Committee for Prevention. Population-based prevention of obesity: the need for comprehensive promotion of healthful eating, physical activity, and energy balance: a scientific statement from American Heart Association Council on Epidemiology and Prevention, Interdisciplinary Committee for Prevention (formerly the expert panel on population and prevention science). Circulation 2008 Jul;118 (4):428–64.

[6] US Centers for Disease control and Prevention. Overweight and obesity. Available at: http://www.cdc.gov/nccdphp/dnpa/obesity/trend/maps/index.htm; 2008. [Accessed 22 October 2009].

[7] Alberti KG, Eckel RH, Grundy SM, Zimmet PZ, Cleeman JI, Donato KA, Fruchart JC, James WP, Loria CM, Smith Jr SC, International Diabetes Federation Task Force on Epidemiology and Prevention., Hational Heart, Lung, and Blood Institute, American Heart Association, World Heart Federation, International Atherosclerosis Society, International Association for the Study of Obesity. Harmonizing the metabolic syndrome: a joint interim statement of the International Diabetes Federation Task Force on Epidemiology and Prevention; National Heart, Lung, and Blood Institute; American Heart Association; World Heart Federation; International Atherosclerosis Society; and International Association for the Study of Obesity. Circulation 2009 Oct;120(16):1640–5.

[8] Alberti KG, Zimmet P, Shaw J, IDF Epidemiology Task Force Consensus Group. The metabolic syndrome—a new worldwide definition. Lancet 2005 Sep;366(9491):1059–62.

[9] Hu FB. Introduction to obesity epidemiology. In: Obesity epidemiology. Oxford University Press; 2008. Chapter 1.

[10] Jain SS, Ramanand SJ, Ramanand JB, Akat PB, Patwardhan MH, Joshi SR. Evaluation of efficacy and safety of orlistat in obese patients. Indian J Endocr Metab 2011 Apr;15(2):99–104.

[11] Brashier DB, Sharma AK, Dahiya N, Singh SK, Khadka A. Lorcaserin: a novel antiobesity drug. J Pharmacol Pharmacother 2014 Apr;5(2):175–8.

[12] Kovač Blaž M, Švab I. A multidisciplinary approach to treating obesity in a community health centre. Zdr Varst 2015 Sep 25;54(4):252–8.

[13] Ma C, Avenell A, Bolland M, Hudson J, Stewart F, Robertson C, Sharma P, Fraser C, MacLennan G. Effects of weight loss interventions for adults who are obese on mortality, cardiovascular disease, and cancer: systematic review and meta-analysis. BMJ 2017 Nov 14;359: j4849. https://doi.org/10.1136/bmj.j4849.

[14] Foster D, Sanchez-Collins S, Cheskin LJ. Multidisciplinary team-based obesity treatment in patients with diabetes: current practices and the state of the science. Diabetes Spectr 2017 Nov; 30(4):244–9. https://doi.org/10.2337/ds17-0045. Erratum in: Diabetes Spectr 2018 Feb; 31(1):119.

[15] Singh GM, Danaei G, Farzadfar F, et al. The age-specific quantitative effects of metabolic risk factors on cardiovascular diseases and diabetes: a pooled analysis. PLoS One 2013;8(7). e65174.

[16] Czernichow S, Kengne AP, Stamatakis E, et al. Bodymass index, waist circumference and waist-hip ratio: which is the better discriminator of cardiovascular disease mortality risk?: evidence from an individual-participant meta-analysis of 82 864 participants from nine cohort studies. Obes Rev 2011;12(9):680–7.

[17] Lauby-Secretan B, Scoccianti C, Loomis D, et al. Body fatness and cancer—viewpoint of the IARC working group. N Engl J Med 2016;375(8):794–8.

[18] Anandacoomarasamy A, Caterson I, Sambrook P, et al. The impact of obesity on the musculoskeletal system. Int J Obes (Lond) 2008;32(2):211–22.

[19] Anstey KJ, Cherbuin N, Budge M, et al. Body mass index in midlife and late-life as a risk factor for dementia: a meta-analysis of prospective studies. Obes Rev 2011;12(5):e426–37.

[20] Kim DD, Basu A. Estimating the medical care costs of obesity in the United States: systematic review, meta-analysis, and empirical analysis. Value Health 2016;19(5):602–13.

[21] von Lengerke T, Krauth C. Economic costs of adult obesity: a review of recent European studies with a focus on subgroup-specific costs. Maturitas 2011;69(3):220–9.

Chapter 2

Study design in obesity epidemiology research

Jacqueline Chu, B.A.[a] and Raman Mehrzad, M.D., M.H.L., M.B.A.[b]
[a]The Ohio State University College of Medicine, Columbus, OH, United States, [b]Department of Plastic and Reconstructive Surgery, Rhode Island Hospital, The Warren Alpert Medical School of Brown University, Providence, RI, United States

Introduction

Obesity is a condition that arises from multiple factors and results in multiple consequences. A useful model for framing the spectrum of obesity epidemiology research can be found in Kim and Popkin (2006) [1]. In this multilevel framework, overweight and obese lie in the middle as the product of many different potential causes and as a cause of many different potential health consequences. Designing research that accurately characterizes the nature of this extremely complex and chronic yet dynamic condition can be a challenging task. This chapter serves as an overview of the major research methods encountered in obesity research and common problems that researchers must be aware of in study design and interpretation.

Research domains in obesity epidemiology

Epidemiology research can be broadly categorized into descriptive, analytic, and experimental. It also reflects a research process that tends to progress from known to unknown. Descriptive epidemiology, as implied by its name, *describes* the nature of the condition of interest—it characterizes the individuals who are affected, the number of people who are affected, the trends of the disease over time, etc. Analytic epidemiology then further assesses for the presence of any causes or effects of the condition of interest. Finally, experimental epidemiology uses the identified causes or consequences to test interventions that can change the course of the condition or its impact on other diseases [2].

Research on obesity epidemiology spans several major domains. Classic descriptive epidemiological research includes large surveillance studies that have been conducted in the United States and other countries that describe

Obesity. https://doi.org/10.1016/B978-0-12-818839-2.00002-8

trends in obesity. For example, the NHANES (National Health and Nutrition Examination Survey) is conducted by the CDC (Centers for Disease Control) yearly. This study, which began in the 1960s, uses surveys and in-person health interviews to collect socioeconomic, lifestyle, and health information from a nationally representative sample of 5000 individuals [3]. In terms of analytic epidemiology, the multilevel framework by Kim and Popkin referenced earlier applies, with extensive research being conducted on both predictors and consequences of obesity. Genome-wide association studies, for example, have been a growing area of research to identify potential genetic predictors of obesity in childhood and adulthood [4–6]. On the other end of the spectrum, much has been written on the link between obesity and the development of cardiovascular disease [7]. Another domain of analytic epidemiology within the field of obesity research focuses on the measures used for obesity, especially the utility and validity of specific body composition measurement tools in defining clinically significant obesity [8]. All this research has been a rich source of hypotheses for experimental epidemiology on effective obesity interventions.

Study designs in obesity epidemiology

In this section, major study designs will be described with examples from the field of obesity epidemiology to highlight the purpose, strengths, and weaknesses of each study method.

The study designs are described based on their order in the hierarchy of determining causality, with descriptive studies like ecological studies being the least able to establish causal relationships between exposure and outcome and randomized controlled trials as the gold standard. Studies higher in the hierarchy are characterized by increased control for confounding variables and increased ability to establish temporality [9]. However, it is important to note that it is still possible to infer causality even without a gold-standard randomized controlled trial, and the criteria that we use to make this inference are called the Bradford Hill criteria [10]. Hill states that nine criteria can be used to evaluate epidemiological data—strength of association, consistency, specificity, temporality, biological gradient, plausibility, coherence, experiment, and analogy. As many aspects of obesity epidemiology would be difficult or even impossible to evaluate using a randomized controlled trial, it becomes important to use these criteria to frame our analysis of obesity epidemiological research.

Descriptive epidemiology

As defined previously, descriptive epidemiology is important for determining trends and patterns for a certain disease. For example, using the data collected by NHANES, the CDC determined that the prevalence of obesity in the United States was 33% in adults and 17% in youth and that this prevalence was stable between 2003 and 2012. Major trends identified by this study were a higher prevalence of obesity in Hispanics and an increased prevalence of obesity in women over 60 [11]. These data allow us to track the disease over time and tell us how we are faring in terms of the disease and in comparison to other countries.

More importantly, these data can serve as a starting point for further analyses regarding potential causes or consequences of disease. One might be interested, for example, in the higher prevalence of obesity in Hispanics and design research to determine causes of this phenomenon and the impact it can have on the health of this population. Indeed, extensive research has been conducted on the social determinants, genetic contributions, and cardiovascular disease and cancer risk associated with obesity in Hispanics [12–15].

Analytic epidemiology

Research on determinants and consequences of obesity lies within the domain of analytic epidemiology. In this category, researchers attempt to find associations and make inferences regarding causation. There are multiple kinds of studies that can be performed, which are described below.

Ecological studies examine population-level data on disease and exposure rates to find any potential associations. The key issues to be aware of when interpreting these studies are confounding and "ecological fallacy."

For example, De Vogli et al. (2011) published an ecological study finding an association between the number of fast food outlets and obesity rates [16]. In this study, the authors compared the obesity prevalence for 26 countries and the number of Subway restaurants available in each of these countries. Data on obesity prevalence were gathered from existing WHO statistics and the number of Subway restaurants was gathered from Subway's website. In addition to calculating the density of Subway restaurants per 100,000 people, the authors also collected data on potential confounding factors that would influence fast food outlet density or obesity prevalence, such as gross national income, proportion living in urban areas, motor vehicles, and Internet users. After adjusting for these confounders, the authors concluded that a higher density of fast food outlets was associated with a higher obesity prevalence. However, even with this data, can we conclude that fast food makes people obese and that we should remove all fast food restaurants? The answer is, of course, no. One can think of many lifestyle, behavioral, or even genetic reasons why countries with higher obesity prevalences also happen to have a greater density of Subway restaurants, even after accounting for the confounders the authors included in this study. As seen in this study, confounding is a major limitation for ecological studies. When examining population-level data with no individual-level data to offer greater granularity, there is very little that can be done to account for the multitude of other factors that impact both the exposure and outcome of interest.

"Ecological fallacy" refers to the concept of misapplying conclusions about populations to individuals within that population. As De Vogli et al. note, their conclusions are not consistent with other research studies on fast food consumption or proximity to fast food restaurants and obesity that use individual-level data. As stated previously, there are a myriad of factors that influence obesity that may differ from individual to individual; the conclusions of an ecological study are not meant to apply to every individual. One can imagine that there are subsets of individuals who may eat fast food every day yet not be obese, and that there are other subsets who do not eat fast food at all but are obese. Therefore, ecological studies, like descriptive epidemiology studies, are not meant to establish causality but to serve as excellent starting points for developing hypotheses appropriate for individual-level research.

Cross-sectional studies

The cross-sectional study design looks for associations at a certain time point. Because these studies are essentially a "snapshot in time," the most important concern with interpreting these studies is the inability to establish temporality, which leads to potential reverse causation.

Marcelina Silva et al. (2018) conducted a cross-sectional study on the association between ultraprocessed food consumption and obesity in Brazil [17]. Variables included in their models were physical activity levels, socioeconomic characteristics, smoking, total energy intake, and nonprocessed food intake. The authors found a positive association between the amount of ultraprocessed food consumed, BMI, and waist circumference, even in individuals with lower total energy intake. This association was seen even after stratification for socioeconomic, demographic, and health characteristics. This study can indicate that ultraprocessed food consumption is a risk factor for obesity and weight gain, but there is always the concern for reverse causation. Perhaps there are behavioral patterns among already obese or overweight individuals that make them prone to select ultraprocessed foods. The directionality of associations found in cross-sectional studies should, therefore, be considered carefully, but these studies can still be valuable as a source of hypotheses for further research.

Case–control studies

Case–control studies compare a group of individuals (cases) with the disease or outcome of interest to a group of individuals who do not (controls). In these studies, there is an exposure or characteristic of interest and, by comparing the levels of this exposure in cases and controls, the study can determine if there is an association between the exposure and the outcome. In addition to concerns of confounding, case–control study design must also consider potential selection biases and recall biases.

Karimbeiki et al. (2018) conducted a case–control study comparing the dietary diversity score (DDS) in overweight or obese adults (cases) and normal-weight adults (controls) in Tehran, Iran [18]. Dietary intake was assessed by a self-administered survey, the Food Frequency Questionnaire, and, on the first visit, the BMI and waist-to-hip ratio were determined. Cases were randomly selected from an obesity treatment group. Controls were randomly selected from volunteers living in Tehran and matched to cases based on socioeconomic status. The authors determined that there was a positive association between the dietary diversity score and obesity. Selection bias, which occurs when the sample population selected is not representative of the general population, is an issue that may affect interpretation of the results of this study. Because cases were selected from an obesity treatment group, these individuals may already be more conscious of their food choices and may try to diversify their diet by including more fruits and vegetables. In addition, the controls were selected and matched to cases based on socioeconomic status, but as a result, the case and control populations differed significantly in terms of age, marital status, and occupation. These factors all play a role in the lifestyle choices that impact weight gain and introduce significant confounding.

Another weakness of case–control studies is the potential for recall biases, which occur when study participants inaccurately report information, but to a differing degree. In Karimbeiki et al., the dietary intake over a week was self-reported in a questionnaire, which could have been completed inaccurately. Investigators attempted to decrease recall bias by having a dietician teach participants how to complete the questionnaire and by collecting data over a week; however, this does not account for the possibility that obese/overweight participants may be more aware of their food habits and respond more accurately. When relying on participants to recall the past, there is always the risk that personal experiences, knowledge, or attentiveness can alter reported information.

The strength of case–control studies lies in their ability to analyze rare outcomes and lower cost in comparison to cohort studies, especially when the study requires assessment of certain genetic variants or biomarkers. For example, Campbell et al. (2010) examined the connection between obesity, colorectal cancer, and tumor microsatellite instability in a case–control study with 1794 case subjects with colorectal cancer and 2684 control subjects, who were unaffected sex-matched siblings [19]. In comparison to obesity, colorectal cancer is a relatively rarer outcome, and there is considerable cost in performing genetic analysis to identify microsatellite instability. A case–control study such as this ensures investigators have a sufficient number of subjects with the desired outcome and cuts down the costs required in running more expensive tests such as gene sequencing.

Case cross-over studies

Case cross-over studies are a type of case–control study in which the case serves as his/her own control. In these types of studies, case individuals are identified and compared to him/herself prior to developing the outcome of interest. This study design, therefore, examines what may have led someone to "cross-over" and become a case. Because this study design necessitates knowing when the outcome developed, it is best suited for acute or abrupt outcomes, for which the onset can be easily identified. Additionally, case cross-over designs are meant to examine proximal causes that immediately led to the outcome, also called "triggers," rather than all potential factors that contributed to the outcome [20]. The most important strength of this study is perfect matching of cases to controls. In addition, because of the short time frame of these studies, changes due to time (i.e., aging, development of chronic diseases, etc.) do not contribute much confounding.

As an example, let us examine a case cross-over study conducted by Woodard et al. (2011) [21]. The authors were interested in whether bariatric surgery led to reduced alcohol metabolism, so they compared blood alcohol content (BAC) and time until sober of patients prior to bariatric surgery to their BAC and time until sober of these same patients at 3 months and 6 months after surgery. BAC and time until sober were determined after consumption of 5 oz of red wine. Both BAC and time until sober were increased in these patients post-bariatric surgery, leading the investigators to conclude that bariatric surgery, the "trigger," indeed led to impaired alcohol metabolism, the "outcome." This study not only highlights the main components of a case cross-over study—a clear and acute onset of the outcome and a proximal cause—but also illustrates the major limitation of this study design, which is that it does not really answer the question of interest. The context of this study is that obese patients who receive bariatric surgery often develop comorbidities associated with alcohol use, including nutritional deficiencies, weight gain, and alcoholism. While this study indicates that bariatric surgery impairs alcohol metabolism and we can infer how that may lead to these comorbidities, this study does not provide that clear link and further research done longitudinally, such as in the form of a prospective cohort study, is still required.

Cohort studies

Cohort studies are in some ways the reverse of a case–control study. Instead of beginning with the outcome and working backward to the exposure, cohort studies begin with individuals who either have the exposure or not and compare the rate of developing the outcome in exposed and nonexposed groups. The prospective cohort study is considered the gold standard in obesity epidemiology research, and much of the following discussion will focus on the strengths and weaknesses of this study type. Prospective cohort studies are at lower risk of selection and recall bias as well as confounding related to reverse causation; however, they tend to be costly and time intensive because they are longitudinal, following participants for potentially decades to assess the development of the outcome of interest. In addition, there are significant challenges in the data collection and statistical analysis of these studies, issues that gain importance as cohort study designs become more and more complex.

As an example, let us examine Kivimäki et al. (2009), a prospective cohort study aimed at identifying association between mental health disorders and obesity [22]. This study used the cohort of the British Whitehall II study, which consisted of London government employees aged 35–55. These 10,308 individuals were followed for 19 years and were assessed for mental health disorders, chronic health conditions, and other behavioral and demographic factors. In addition, weight and height were directly measured. These assessments were conducted at four different time points spaced roughly every 6 years. This study demonstrates the ability of prospective cohort studies to establish temporality through repeated measures of the variables of interest and through long-term follow-up. The authors of this study were, therefore, able to assess the directionality (and assess the possibility of reverse causation) of obesity and mental health disorders. They found that common mental disorders predicted subsequent obesity and that the risk of obesity increased with the number of assessments that demonstrated common mental disorders. Of note, this relationship was only seen with individuals with a common mental disorder at the baseline assessment.

In addition to determining directionality, this study capitalized on another strength of using repeated measures and long-term follow-up by establishing dose–response relationships between the number of assessments positive for obesity and the number of assessments positive for a common mental disorder. By doing so, the authors accounted for the potential of both mental disorders and obesity to fluctuate over time. When the tested exposures can change over the study period, such that an obese individual at baseline can lose weight and become normal weight or a person with depression may seek treatment and be in remission, it may not be appropriate to use one measure of weight or mental health taken at the beginning or end of a study period, as this may not actually quantify the true level of these exposures in the studied individual over the entire study period.

The prospective cohort study design is not without weaknesses. For example, the above study suffered from substantial loss to follow-up, from 10,175 subjects at phase 1 to 4363 subjects actually included in the primary statistical analysis. There is potential selection bias as there may be certain characteristics that may make an individual inclined to discontinue participation in the study or fail to respond to certain components of the study. In order to account for this missing data, one can remove all participants without complete follow-up from statistical analysis, as was done in this study, and analyze for differences between participants who were included and excluded. However, in smaller studies, this may substantially lower the power of the analysis. Another method is multiple imputation, in which researchers fill in missing values to create multiple complete datasets, which are then each individually analyzed and compared to the other datasets [23].

One additional strength of cohort studies is the ability to conduct nested case–control studies without some of the selection bias issues that a classic case–control study encounters. In this study design, a sample of the cases and matched group of controls is selected from an existing cohort study. For example, Agnoli et al. (2010), conducted a nested case–control study using the ORDET cohort to analyze the association between metabolic syndrome and postmenopausal breast cancer [24]. In this study, the 181 women who developed new breast cancer and matched controls were selected out of 3966 postmenopausal women in the ORDET cohort. As the subjects chosen for the case–control study were part of a predefined cohort, there is no risk of selection bias. This study design is excellent for comparing biomarkers that would be costly to assess for the entire cohort. Agnoli et al., for example, measured triglycerides, HDL-cholesterol, and glucose for cases and controls using existing serum samples taken from the entire cohort at the baseline.

Experimental epidemiology

The ultimate goal of any analytical epidemiological research is to identify potential targets for intervention. Recognizing that obesity and cardiovascular disease are linked, for example, may trigger one to think about what can be done to prevent cardiovascular disease in obese patients or to consider the effectiveness of treating obesity for the treatment of cardiovascular disease. The gold standard for this type of research is the randomized controlled trial (RCT). However, it may not be feasible or ethical to conduct an RCT for all types of interventions, so many types of non-RCT intervention studies exist as well. The following section will describe some strengths and weaknesses of these experimental study designs.

Randomized controlled trials

The design of a randomized controlled trial is evident in its name. Participants are randomly assigned to either an experimental group, which receives the intervention being studied, or a control group, which receives no intervention. In theory, there is no selection bias and all confounding patient characteristics are accounted for by randomizing the group assignment process. Because of this, RCTs should be able to establish the causal role of the studied exposure variable without the concern of confounding variables impacting the studied outcome. However, in practice, RCTs have their own methodological issues that affect investigators' ability to make definitive conclusions.

One of the most important threats to the validity of an RCT is dropout—participants fail to complete the full trial. A systematic review by Moroshko et al. (2011) found that attrition rates for weight loss interventions varied from 10% to 80% [25]. This introduces significant risk of selection bias to the study, as individuals who decide to remain in the study may differ from those who do not. Indeed, studies on attrition rates have demonstrated differences in baseline BMI, age, gender, ethnicity, education levels, mental health, and weight-loss expectations between those who remain in the RCT and those who do not, all factors that can play a significant role in participants' abilities to manage their weight or benefit from weight loss interventions [25, 26]. Randomized controlled studies with high attrition rates should therefore be interpreted with caution, as their results may merely be a reflection of the population they studied.

Nonadherence can similarly affect the conclusions of RCTs. For example, a retrospective study by Martin et al. (2018) of the participants of an RCT on daily self-weighing (DSW) and daily activity tracking (DAT) in African American breast cancer survivors found that weight gain and weight fluctuation were associated with periods of nonadherence to DSW and DAT [27]. Failing to account for nonadherence in this randomized controlled study could result in underestimating the effect of the intervention, with less overall weight loss recorded due to nonadherence negating some of the weight loss that occurred during periods of adherence. However, it is important to consider that 100% adherence is unexpected in real life. Therefore, while the true effect of the intervention may be underestimated, this underestimated effect may actually have more external validity and be more reflective of how this intervention may play out in the "real world."

Non-RCT studies

There are instances when conducting an RCT on a particular intervention may not be feasible, so a nonrandomized method is used. For example, Kain et al. (2004) conducted a school-based obesity prevention intervention involving nutrition education for children and patients, healthier snacks, and increased physical activity [28]. The authors note that randomization of school sites was not possible as the funding was from the Chilean government, so government education officials chose schools that they felt most needed the intervention, potentially resulting in an intervention population with a higher prevalence of obesity. In addition, one can imagine the enormous costs, in terms of both time and money, associated with an intervention like this. The investigators of this study needed to hire full-time nutritionists for 6 months, alter school schedules to accommodate increased physical activity, and communicate with food vendors to change provided snack options. Randomization may not necessarily work for interventions at this scale, as it requires extensive buy-in from the communities selected and not every community may be interested in implementing such a project.

Sometimes it is unethical to conduct an RCT. For example, Benizri et al. (2013) conducted a prospective nonrandomized controlled study comparing robotic gastric bypass to the standard of care, laparoscopic gastric bypass [29]. The study aimed to compare perioperative outcomes and complications for the two procedures and found that while the robotic procedure reduced operative time, it also had higher complication rates and longer hospital stays. This study cannot be conducted in a randomized manner as patients should ethically have a choice of which procedure they want, especially when one procedure may have increased risk of harm.

The future of research in obesity epidemiology

Much work is still being done to improve the quality and usefulness of research in obesity epidemiology. Recently, the NIH produced a set of recommendations regarding research directions in obesity as part of their Pathways to Prevention (P2P) Workshop [30]. One key gap that they recognized was the lack of standardization in data reporting, including research definitions and research measures. This results in duplicative, inefficient efforts regarding data collection and the use of measurement tools, such as questionnaires, that have poor comparability or validity. This is a particularly important issue for multicenter or pooled cohort studies, which combine cohorts from diverse populations. For example, in a pooled cohort study performed by Lu et al. (2014) examining the metabolic factors in obesity that contribute to coronary heart disease, the authors recognized that some of the limitations of their study included inconsistent measurements of mediators, incomplete reporting of certain outcomes, and inaccessibility of certain cohort datasets [31]. The contributors of the NIH P2P Workshop contend that issues such as these can be avoided through increased communication among researchers, policymakers, and funding sources to produce integrated databases using a common library for definitions and measures. They argue that this increased collaboration can also contribute to the production of research outcomes and measures that are important to policymakers, such as cost effectiveness and population impact [30]. A good example of a study that incorporated these metrics is that from Gortmaker et al. (2015), which conducted a cost-effectiveness analysis of four obesity interventions [32].

In addition, they advocate for the increased use of new technologies that can provide more objective measurements and more accurate data collection [30]. Information gathered using smart phone applications or wearable technologies can improve the accuracy of dietary intake or physical activity measures that have historically been measured using questionnaires or interviews, which are prone to recall biases [33].

Finally, with the complexity of prospective cohort studies and the need to adjust for many confounding subject characteristics, ensure sufficient sample size without selection bias, and account for losses to follow up, among other issues, the statistics analytical skills required to properly conduct these studies are increasing. The need for increased statistical support or training for obesity epidemiology researchers is recognized by many in the field [23, 30, 34].

References

[1] Kim S, Popkin BM. Commentary: understanding the epidemiology of overweight and obesity—a real global public health concern. Int J Epidemiol 2006;35(1):60–7. Available from: http://academic.oup.com/ije/article/35/1/60/849921/Commentary-Understanding-the-epidemiology-of.

[2] Arnett DK, Claas SA. Introduction to epidemiology. In: Clinical and translational science: principles of human research. 2nd ed. Elsevier Inc.; 2017. p. 53–69.

[3] CDC. NHANES—about the National Health and Nutrition Examination Survey. CDC; 2017. Available from: https://www.cdc.gov/nchs/nhanes/about_nhanes.htm.

[4] Loos RJF, Yeo GSH. The bigger picture of FTO—the first GWAS-identified obesity gene. Nat Rev Endocrinol 2014;10(1):51–61.

[5] Zhao J, Bradfield JP, Zhang H, et al. Role of BMI-associated loci identified in GWAS meta-analyses in the context of common childhood obesity in European Americans. Obesity 2011;19 (12):2436–9. https://doi.org/10.1038/oby.2011.237.

[6] Wang J, Mei H, Chen W, et al. Study of eight GWAS-identified common variants for association with obesity-related indices in Chinese children at puberty. Int J Obes (Lond) 2012;36 (4):542–7.

[7] Reis JP, Loria CM, Lewis CE, et al. Association between duration of overall and abdominal obesity beginning in young adulthood and coronary artery calcification in middle age. JAMA 2013;310(3):280–8.

[8] Jayawardena R, Ranasinghe P, Ranathunga T, Mathangasinghe Y, Wasalathanththri S, Hills AP. Novel anthropometric parameters to define obesity and obesity-related disease in adults: a systematic review. Nutr Rev 2019; https://doi.org/10.1093/nutrit/nuz078/5678778.

[9] Stephenson JM, Babiker A. Overview of study design in clinical epidemiology. Sex Transm Infect 2000;76(4):244–7.

[10] Fedak KM, Bernal A, Capshaw ZA, Gross S. Applying the Bradford Hill criteria in the 21st century: how data integration has changed causal inference in molecular epidemiology. Emerg Themes Epidemiol 2015;12(1).

[11] Ogden CL, Carroll MD, Kit BK, Flegal KM. Prevalence of childhood and adult obesity in the United States, 2011–2012. JAMA 2014;311(8):806–14.

[12] Liu J, Probst JC, Harun N, Bennett KJ, Torres ME. Acculturation, physical activity, and obesity among Hispanic adolescents. Ethn Health 2009;14(5):509–25.

[13] Comuzzie AG, Cole SA, Laston SL, et al. Novel genetic loci identified for the pathophysiology of childhood obesity in the hispanic population. PLoS One 2012;7(12) e51954. Available from: https://dx.plos.org/10.1371/journal.pone.0051954.

[14] Smith TM, Colón-Ramos U, Pinard CA, Yaroch AL. Household food insecurity as a determinant of overweight and obesity among low-income Hispanic subgroups: data from the 2011–2012 California Health Interview Survey. Appetite 2016;97:37–42.

[15] Aballay LR, Eynard AR, Díaz Mdel P, Navarro A, Muñoz SE. Overweight and obesity: a review of their relationship to metabolic syndrome, cardiovascular disease, and cancer in South America. Nutr Rev 2013;71(3):168–79.

[16] de Vogli R, Kouvonen A, Gimeno D. "Globesization": ecological evidence on the relationship between fast food outlets and obesity among 26 advanced economies. Crit Public Health 2011;21(4):395–402.

[17] Marcelina Silva F, Giatti L, Carvalho de Figueiredo R, et al. Consumption of ultra-processed food and obesity: cross sectional results from the Brazilian Longitudinal Study of Adult Health (ELSA-Brasil) cohort 2008–2010. Public Health Nutr 2018;21(12):2271–9.

[18] Karimbeiki R, Pourmasoumi M, Feizi A, et al. Higher dietary diversity score is associated with obesity: a case–control study. Public Health 2018;157:127–34.
[19] Campbell PT, Jacobs ET, Ulrich CM, et al. Case–control study of overweight, obesity, and colorectal cancer risk, overall and by tumor microsatellite instability status. JNCI 2010;102 (6):391–400. Available from: https://academic.oup.com/jnci/article-lookup/doi/10.1093/jnci/djq011.
[20] Maclure M, Mittleman MA. Should we use a case-crossover design? Annu Rev Public Health 2000;21(1):193–221. Available from:http://www.annualreviews.org/doi/10.1146/annurev.publhealth.21.1.193.
[21] Woodard GA, Downey J, Hernandez-Boussard T, Morton JM. Impaired alcohol metabolism after gastric bypass surgery: a case-crossover trial. J Am Coll Surg 2011;212(2):209–14.
[22] Kivimäki M, Lawlor DA, Singh-Manoux A, et al. Common mental disorder and obesity-insight from four repeat measures over 19 years: prospective Whitehall II cohort study. BMJ 2009;339(7726):902–5.
[23] George BJ, Beasley TM, Brown AW, et al. Common scientific and statistical errors in obesity research. Obesity 2016;24(4):781–90. https://doi.org/10.1002/oby.21449.
[24] Agnoli C, Berrino F, Abagnato CA, et al. Metabolic syndrome and postmenopausal breast cancer in the ORDET cohort: a nested case-control study. Nutr Metab Cardiovasc Dis 2010;20 (1):41–8.
[25] Moroshko I, Brennan L, O'Brien P. Predictors of dropout in weight loss interventions: a systematic review of the literature. Obes Rev 2011;12(11):912–34. https://doi.org/10.1111/j.1467-789X.2011.00915.x.
[26] Kaiser KA, Affuso O, Desmond R, Allison DB. Baseline participant characteristics and risk for dropout from 10 obesity randomized controlled trials: a pooled analysis of individual level data. Front Nutr 2014;1:.
[27] Martin CL, Tate DF, Valle CG. Nonadherence to daily self-weighing and activity tracking is associated with weight fluctuations among African American breast cancer survivors. PLoS One 2018;13(6) e0199751. Available from: https://dx.plos.org/10.1371/journal.pone.0199751.
[28] Kain J, Uauy R, Albala, Vio F, Cerda R, Leyton B. School-based obesity prevention in Chilean primary school children: methodology and evaluation of a controlled study. Int J Obes (Lond) 2004;28(4):483–93.
[29] Benizri EI, Renaud M, Reibel N, et al. Perioperative outcomes after totally robotic gastric bypass: a prospective nonrandomized controlled study. Am J Surg 2013;206(2):145–51.
[30] Emmons KM, Doubeni CA, Fernandez ME, Miglioretti DL, Samet JM. National institutes of health pathways to prevention workshop: methods for evaluating natural experiments in obesity. Ann Intern Med 2018;168(11):809–14.
[31] Lu Y, Hajifathalian K, Ezzati M, et al. Metabolic mediators of the effects of body-mass index, overweight, and obesity on coronary heart disease and stroke: a pooled analysis of 97 prospective cohorts with 1·8 million participants. Lancet 2014;383(9921):970–83. Available from: https://linkinghub.elsevier.com/retrieve/pii/S014067361361836X.
[32] Gortmaker SL, Long MW, Resch SC, et al. Cost effectiveness of childhood obesity interventions: evidence and methods for CHOICES. Am J Prev Med 2015;49(1):102–11.
[33] Timmins KA, Green MA, Radley D, Morris MA, Pearce J. How has big data contributed to obesity research? A review of the literature. Int J Obes (Lond) 2018;42(12):1951–62.
[34] Sallis JF, Story M, Lou D. Study designs and analytic strategies for environmental and policy research on obesity, physical activity, and diet. Recommendations from a meeting of experts. Am. J Prev Med 2009;36(2 Suppl):S72–7.

Chapter 3

Prevalence and trends in obesity in the United States and affluent countries

Ollin Venegas, B.A. and Raman Mehrzad, M.D., M.H.L., M.B.A.
Department of Plastic and Reconstructive Surgery, Rhode Island Hospital, The Warren Alpert Medical School of Brown University, Providence, RI, United States

Introduction

According to recent studies on the trends of BMI worldwide, the prevalence of obesity has doubled in more than 80 countries since 1980 [1, 2]. Moreover, nearly every country—excluding parts of sub-Saharan Africa and Asia—has observed an increase in obesity every year since 1975 [3]. Worldwide, 10.8% of adult males and 14.8% of adult females have obesity (Fig. 1 and Table 1) [4]. Overall, this represents 3.4- and 2.3-fold increases in obesity in adult males and females, respectively, in 40 years [4]. However, these trends are heterogeneous across countries with regard to the steepness of increase. The prevalence of a BMI $\geq$30 varies by country from <3.0% in Vietnam to >58% in the Micronesian island of Nauru [3, 5]. This wide range reflects the economic, environmental, ethnic, and social differences throughout the world. Moreover, the tabulation of the prevalence of obesity in each country is not conducted annually, as in the United States and other high-income countries. As a result, this chapter will focus on the trends of obesity in the United States and other affluent countries—defined in this chapter as the top 25 countries according to gross national income (Fig. 2 and Table 2) [6].

Measuring prevalence

In ideal conditions, the prevalence of obesity would be measured via a classification system that had the following characteristics: (1) based on a practical measurement widely available to providers regardless of their setting; (2) accurately predict health risk (prognosis); and (3) used to assign treatment strategies and goals [7]. The most accurate ways to measure body fat—the major component

Obesity. https://doi.org/10.1016/B978-0-12-818839-2.00003-X

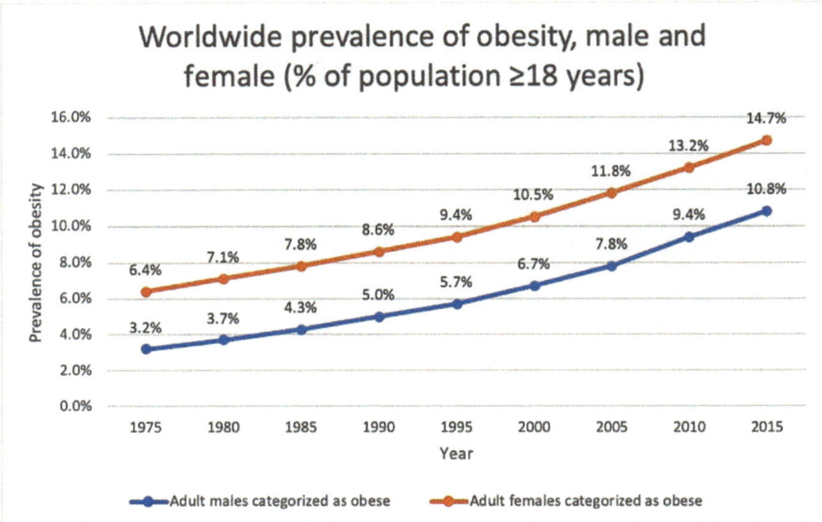

FIG. 1 Change in prevalence of obesity over time. Percentage of adults defined as obese, worldwide, has increased substantially since 1975. *Adapted from Gender Statistics, The World Bank.*

TABLE 1 Worldwide prevalence of obesity, male and female (% of population ≥ 18 years).

Year	Percentage of males categorized as obese	Percentage of females categorized as obese
1975	3.2	6.4
1980	3.7	7.1
1985	4.3	7.8
1990	5.0	8.6
1995	5.7	9.4
2000	6.7	10.5
2005	7.8	11.8
2010	9.4	13.2
2015	10.8	14.7

Adapted from Gender Statistics, The World Bank.

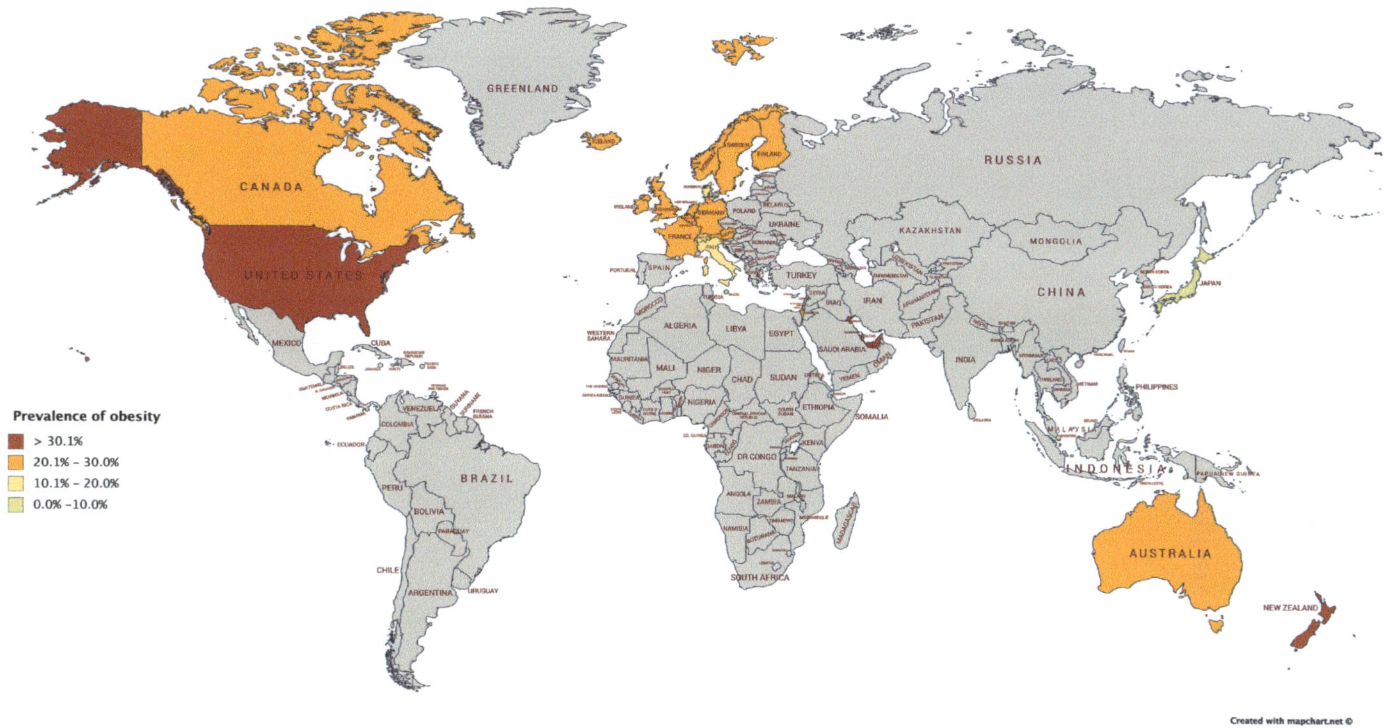

FIG. 2 Prevalence of obesity in US and affluent countries. Percentage of adults defined as obese among top 25 countries according to gross national income (GNI). Most recent data. *Adapted from WHO, Global Health Observatory*.

TABLE 2 Prevalence of obesity in the United States and affluent countries in 2016.

Top 25 countries per GNI (alphabetical order)	Prevalence of obesity among adults (%)
Australia	29.0
Austria	20.1
Belgium	22.1
Canada	29.4
Denmark	19.7
Finland	22.2
France	21.6
Germany	22.3
Iceland	21.9
Ireland	25.3
Israel	26.1
Italy	19.9
Japan	4.3
Kuwait	37.9
Luxembourg	22.6
Netherlands	20.4
New Zealand	30.8
Norway	23.1
Qatar	35.1
Singapore	6.1
Sweden	20.6
Switzerland	19.5
United Arab Emirates	31.7
United Kingdom	27.8
United States	36.2

Adapted from WHO, Global Health Observatory—body mass index (BMI); prevalence of obesity among adults, BMI $\geq$30, age-standardized; estimates by country; year 2016; World Development Indicators, The World Bank; GNI per capita (current US$).

of body weight responsible for adverse health outcomes—are imaging modalities and indirect measuring [7]. The imaging studies include dual-energy x-ray absorptiometry (DEXA) scans, computed tomography (CT), and magnetic resonance imaging (MRI). Indirect measurements include underwater weighing, air displacement (BODPOD), or bioimpedance analysis (BIA). However, these systems are impractical and cost-prohibitive in everyday clinical encounters and are utilized for research purposes. As a result, body mass index (BMI) is the most widely used standard for classifying the somatic type.

Under the BMI classification (Table 3), normal weight is defined as ≥18.5–24.9 kg/m [2], overweight as ≥25.0–29.9 kg/m^2, and obese as ≥30 kg/m^2 [8]. Obesity is then subdivided into three classes: Class I is defined as 30.0–34.9 kg/m^2, Class II as 35.0–39.9 kg/m^2, and Class III (severe obesity) as >40.0 kg/m^2 [8].

In the United States, prevalence data on obesity has been collected in two ways: (1) Annual telephone surveys conducted by the Departments of Health in all 50 states and aggregated into the Behavior Risk Factor Surveillance System (BRFSS) by the Centers for Disease Control and Prevention (CDC); (2) Country-wide field surveys conducted in participants' homes and standardized physical exams in mobile examination centers by the National Center for Health Statistics, known as the National Health and Nutrition Survey (NHANES). Similar national health surveys are conducted in all affluent countries as well.

Past trends

The role of socioeconomic status in the obesity pandemic has shifted over the past century. Until the turn of the 20th century, obesity in the United States and

TABLE 3 Classification of body mass index (BMI).

Classification	BMI (kg/m^2)	Obesity class
Underweight	<18.5	–
Normal weight	18.5–24.9	–
Overweight	25.0–29.9	–
Obese	30.0–34.9	I
	35.0–39.9	II
Severe obesity[a]	≥40.0	III

[a]*Class III has also been referred to as extreme, massive, or morbid obesity. The authors refrained from the use of these descriptors in efforts to reduce the perpetuation of weight stigma and bias.*
Adapted from Executive summary. Obes Res 1998;6:51S–179S. https://doi.org/10.1002/j.1550-8528.1998.tb00690.x.

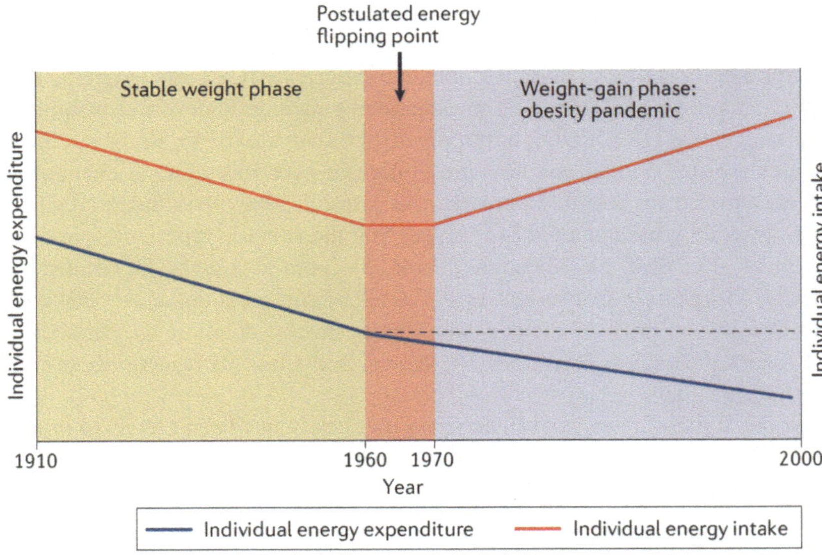

FIG. 3 The energy flipping point. Food intake (*red*) and energy expenditure (*blue*) in the United States between 1910 and 2000. From 1910 to ~1960, energy expenditure was reduced owing to technical changes in the workplace and growing motorization. This reduction in energy expenditure was matched by a parallel reduction in energy intake and resulted in a stable weight phase. Owing to an increase in the production of energy-dense, carbohydrate-rich, and fat-rich foods in the United States around the early 1970s, an energy "flipping point" marks the beginning of the weight-gain phase, in which increased energy intake was disproportional to either plateauing (*dashed line*) or further decreasing energy expenditure demands (accurate measurements of energy expenditure are unavailable) [10].

Europe was directly associated with income. Individuals with more income were more likely to be overweight or obese. It has been postulated that in most high-income countries, the energy balance at the population level is characterized by an energy "flipping point" (Fig. 3). For the United States and other high-income countries, this occurred during the 1960s and 1970s when the food supply for refined carbohydrates and fat markedly increased. This also coincided with a reduction in home cooking, increased affordability/prevalence of home appliances (refrigerators, televisions, air conditioners, etc.) in households, reduced physical activity, exponential growth in computer-based work, and more persuasive food marketing.

Prevalence of obesity in adults

For 2017–18, the age-adjusted prevalence of obesity among US adults aged 20 and over was 42.4%, and 9.2% had severe obesity [9]. Overall, this represents an 84% increase in prevalence from 23.0% in 2001–the first year this statistic was included in the National Health Interview Survey (NHIS) results [10]. Based on US Census data of adults aged 20 or over from 2001, this 84% increase equals the addition of approximately 52.7 million US adults categorized as obese, or nearly 6.5 times the population of New York City in 2001 [11, 12]. When divided into age brackets, the prevalence was 40.0% among young adults (aged 20–39), 44.8% among middle-aged adults (aged 40–59), and 42.8% among older adults (aged 60 and over) [9].

When further separated by sex, the prevalence of obesity in men and women was statistically similar (Fig. 4). Among men, the prevalence was 40.3% among those aged 20–39, 46.4% among those aged 40–59, and 42.2% among those aged 60 and over [9]. With women, the prevalence was 39.7% among those age 20–39, 43.3% among those aged 40–59, and 43.3 among those aged 60 and over [9].

However, the increase in the prevalence was not uniformly distributed across all 50 states, much less across counties, cities, or neighborhoods/wards. Obesity is a multifactorial problem resulting from a combination of individual, community, and geographic influences [13–15]. Geographic disparities in obesity prevalence have been documented and associated with demographic, urbanization, socioeconomic, health care, and environmental factors [15, 16].

According to the authors' analysis of the 2018 BRFSS data, the obesity prevalence significantly varied from region to region (Northeast, South, Midwest, and West), division to division, and state to state. Overall, the prevalence of obesity was lowest in the Pacific and New England (27.8% and 28.1%, respectively) and the highest in the West South Central and East South Central (35.9% and 36.7%) (Fig. 5 and Table 4). Among younger adults (aged 18–44), obesity was lowest in the Pacific (27.1%), highest in the West South Central and East

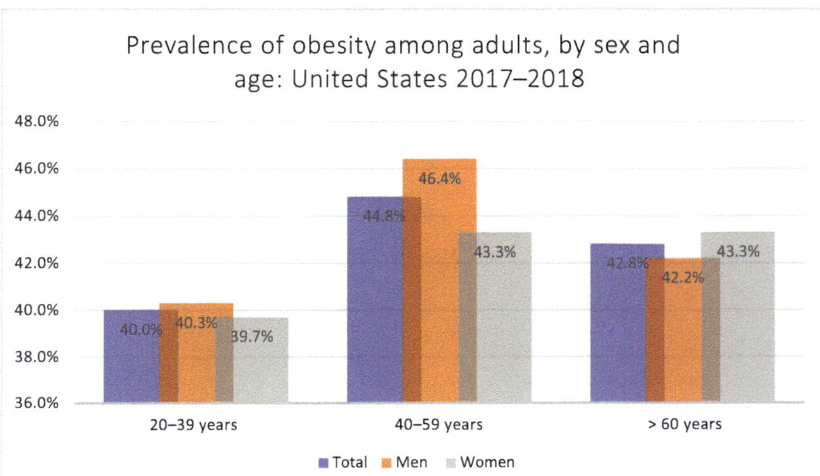

FIG. 4 Prevalence of obesity among adults in the United States. *Adapted from Hales CM, Carroll MD, Fryar CD, Ogden CL. Prevalence of obesity and severe obesity among adults: United States, 2017–2018. NCHS Data Brief, no 360. Hyattsville, MD: National Center for Health Statistics. 2020.*

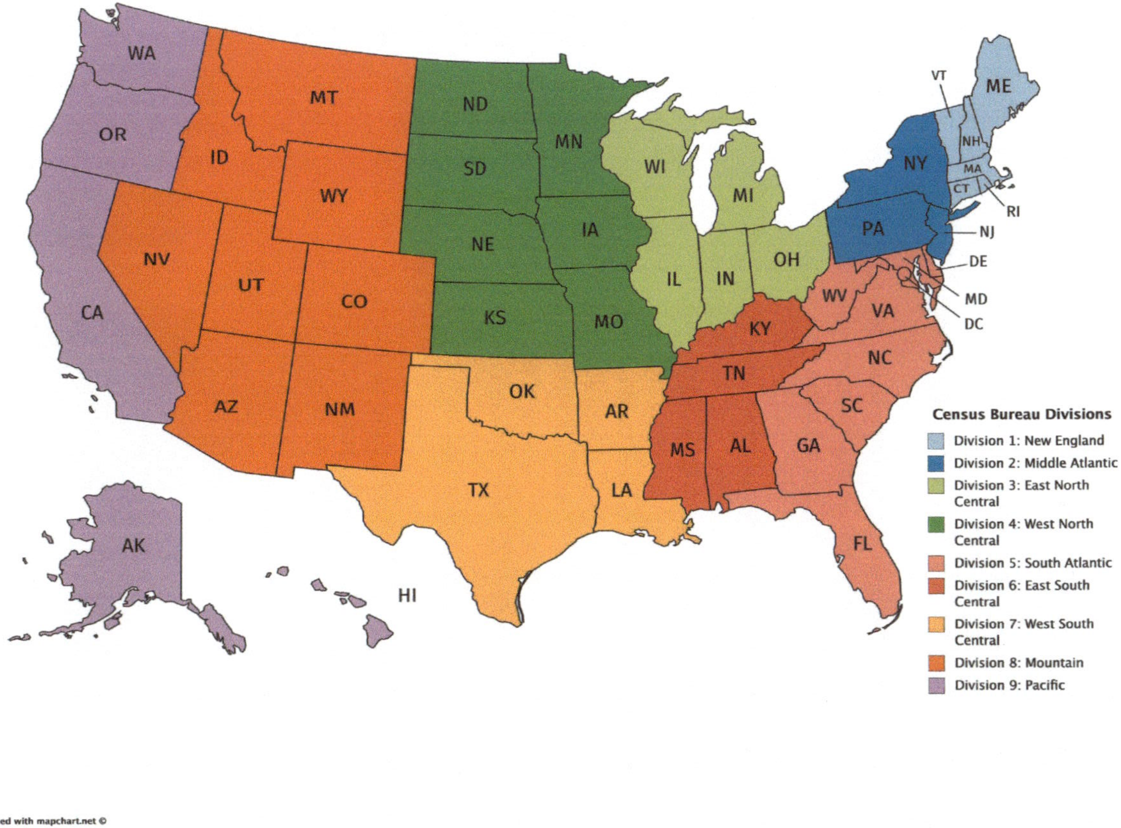

FIG. 5 Census Bureau Divisions of the United States. *Adapted from Division Map, data.census.gov, https://www2.census.gov/geo/pdfs/maps-data/maps/reference/us_regdiv.pdf.*

TABLE 4 Prevalence of obesity by US Census Divisions, 2018.

Division (alphabetical order)	Prevalence of obesity (%)
East North Central	33.0
East South Central	36.7
Middle Atlantic	28.1
Mountain	28.3
New England	28.1
Pacific	27.8
South Atlantic	32.2
West North Central	33.4
West South Central	35.9

Adapted from BRFSS 2018, Table of overweight and obesity; BMI.

South Central (35.6% and 36.9%), and similar in all other divisions (range 27.4–33.3%). Among older adults (≥45), obesity was lowest in the Pacific division (27.3%), and highest in the East South Central (≥38%) (Table 5). Regionally, the South and Midwest consistently have the highest prevalences at 33.2% and 34.1%, respectively. The Northeast and West tied for third place at 28.1%. These findings were consistent with the results of other studies [13–16]. Finally, all states had more than 20% of adults with obesity (Fig. 6 and Table 6). Colorado and Hawaii had the lowest prevalence at 23.0% and 24.9%, respectively [17]. Mississippi and West Virginia were tied for the highest prevalence at 39.5%, followed by Kentucky at 36.6% [17].

The reasons for these geographic patterns are complex, involving innumerable aspects of community features such as the natural environment, access to recreational facilities and health care, the ratio of food outlets to fast food restaurants, the history of residential segregation, the rates of unemployment, the percentage living at or below federal poverty thresholds, the percentage of uninsured, the mean age of the population, the percentage of families headed by single mothers, and the highest level of educational attainment per household. Nevertheless, understanding the interdependence of these factors and the subsequent influence on the prevalence of obesity has been the subject of investigation over the past decade.

In the West and Midwest, the impact of an unemployed labor force was significantly related to higher obesity prevalence compared to all other regions, including the South where unemployment is among the highest in the nation. Interestingly, the positive association between physical inactivity and obesity

TABLE 5 **Prevalence of obesity by US Census Divisions and age groups, 2018.**

Division (alphabetical order)	Prevalence of obesity (%) for younger adults (aged 18–44)	Prevalence of obesity (%) for older adults (aged >45)
East North Central	33.0	33.1
East South Central	36.7	36.8
Middle Atlantic	28.1	27.9
Mountain	28.3	28.0
New England	28.1	27.5
Pacific	27.8	27.3
South Atlantic	32.2	31.7
West North Central	33.4	33.1
West South Central	35.9	35.3

Adapted from BRFSS 2018, Table of overweight and obesity; BMI.

prevalence was significantly weaker in the Midwest in comparison to the other regions. The reason for this regional distinction is unclear.

In the South, residential segregation between impoverished and wealthy populations was significantly linked to lower obesity prevalence. Moreover, black populations were linked to higher rates of obesity. This relationship was strongest in the South compared to other regions. One other notable finding is that the greatest concentration of adult obesity in the country is clustered in a large contiguous region of counties in the South that spans Alabama, Mississippi, Louisiana, and Arkansas.

One measure of health care context that held significance across all regions was physician density. This metric was negatively correlated with obesity prevalence in all areas of the country. This highlights the increasing demand for physician supply in medically underserved areas. Finally, of note, there are factors that have not been found statistically significant across all regions, including food environment indicators and comparisons between urban and rural areas.

Differences in the prevalence of obesity among adults by race and Hispanic origin have been a topic of contentious debate over the decades. Historically, minorities have been disproportionately affected by noncommunicable, chronic diseases (diabetes, heart disease) in comparison to those identifying as white. The 2017–18 NHANES results found some data on these differences

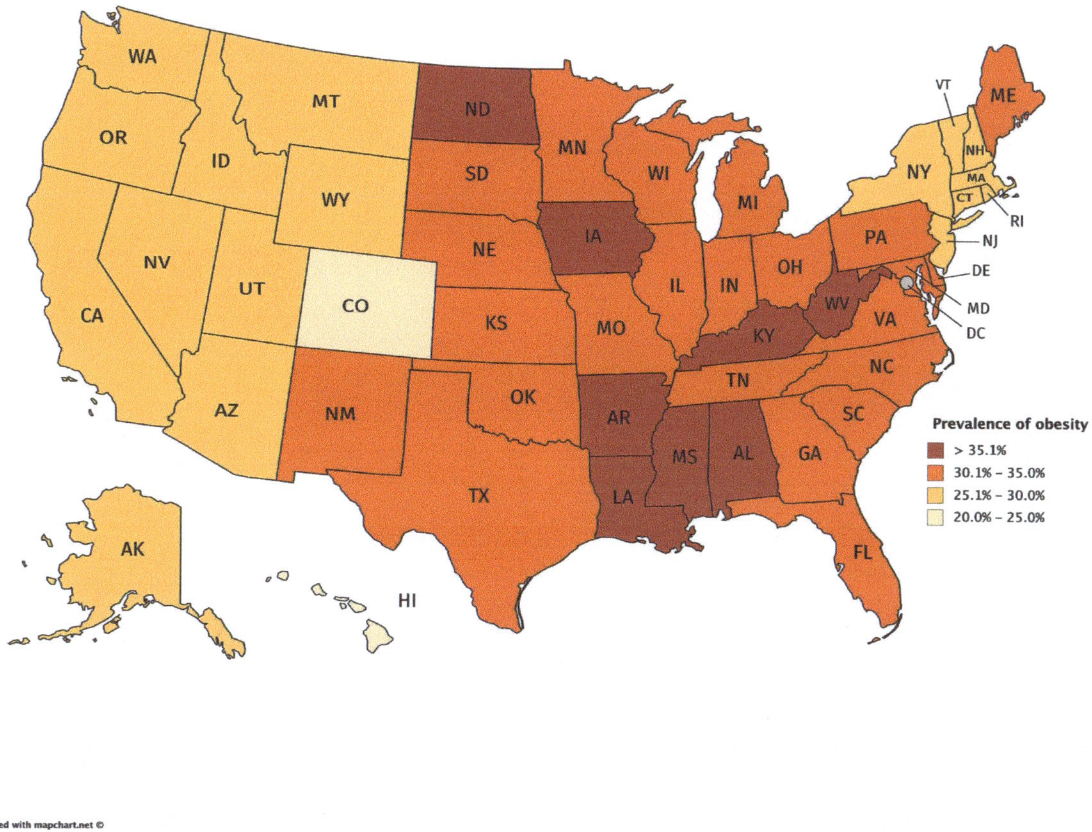

FIG. 6 Prevalence of obesity in the United States in 2018. *Adapted from Adult obesity prevalence maps 2018, Centers for Disease Control and Prevention.*

TABLE 6 Prevalence of obesity in the 50 states in 2018.

States (alphabetical order)	Prevalence of obesity (%) of state population
Alabama	36.2
Alaska	29.5
Arizona	29.5
Arkansas	37.1
California	25.8
Colorado	23.0
Connecticut	27.4
Delaware	33.5
Florida	30.7
Georgia	32.5
Hawaii	24.9
Idaho	28.4
Illinois	31.8
Indiana	34.1
Iowa	35.3
Kansas	34.4
Kentucky	36.6
Louisiana	36.8
Maine	30.4
Maryland	30.9
Massachusetts	25.7
Michigan	33.0
Minnesota	30.1
Mississippi	39.5
Missouri	35.0
Montana	26.9
Nebraska	34.1
Nevada	29.5
New Hampshire	29.6
New Jersey	25.7

TABLE 6 Prevalence of obesity in the 50 states in 2018.—cont'd

States (alphabetical order)	Prevalence of obesity (%) of state population
New Mexico	32.3
New York	27.6
North Carolina	33.0
North Dakota	35.1
Ohio	34.0
Oklahoma	34.8
Oregon	29.9
Pennsylvania	30.9
Rhode Island	27.7
South Carolina	34.3
South Dakota	30.1
Tennessee	34.4
Texas	34.8
Utah	27.8
Vermont	27.5
Virginia	30.4
Washington	28.7
West Virginia	39.5
Wisconsin	32.0
Wyoming	29.0

Adapted from Adult obesity prevalence maps 2018, Centers for Disease Control and Prevention.

(Table 7). Non-Hispanic blacks had the highest prevalence of obesity (49.6%) in comparison to all other race and Hispanic origin groups. Non-Hispanic Asian adults had the lowest prevalence of obesity (17.4%) compared with non-Hispanic whites (42.2%) and Hispanic (44.8%) adults.

Moreover, non-Hispanic black women had the highest prevalence (56.9%) over all other groups by a margin of 11%. The prevalence was the lowest in non-Hispanic Asian women (17.2%) compared with non-Hispanic white (39.8%) and Hispanic (43.7%).

TABLE 7 Prevalence of obesity among adults by demographic factors: United States.

Sex, race, and ethnicity	Prevalence of obesity (%)
Men, Hispanic	45.7
Men, non-Hispanic Asian	17.2
Men, non-Hispanic black	41.1
Men, non-Hispanic white	44.7
Women, Hispanic	43.7
Women, non-Hispanic Asian	17.5
Women, non-Hispanic black	56.9
Women, non-Hispanic white	39.8

Adapted from Hales CM, Carroll MD, Fryar CD, Ogden CL. Prevalence of obesity and severe obesity among adults: United States, 2017–2018. NCHS Data Brief, no 360. Hyattsville, MD: National Center for Health Statistics; 2020.

Interestingly, no significant differences were found among men across race and Hispanic-origin groups. The prevalence was lowest in non-Hispanic Asian (17.5%) compared with non-Hispanic white (44.7%), non-Hispanic black (41.1%), and Hispanic (45.7%) men.

Finally, non-Hispanic black adults had the highest prevalence of severe obesity at 13.8% while non-Hispanic Asian adults had the lowest at 2.0% [9]. Women had a higher prevalence of severe obesity (11.5%) than men (6.9%) [9]. Among the age brackets, adults aged 40–59 had the highest prevalence (11.5%), followed by aged 20–39 (9.1%), and aged 60 and over (5.8%) [9]. Overall, the age-adjusted prevalence among adults in the United States was 9.2% [9].

Some studies have shown a relationship between obesity prevalence and socioeconomic status measured as educational level or income. The results for the most part were only able to show a weak association. The CDC last analyzed this relationship in 2010. Three key findings were made. First, that among men, obesity prevalence was generally similar across all educational and income levels, with a tendency to be slightly higher at higher incomes. However, among non-Hispanic black and Mexican American men, those with a higher income were more likely to be obese than those with a lower income [18].

Next, among women, obesity prevalence increased as income and education decreased. Out of the women surveyed who lived in households with income below the poverty level, 42.0% were obese, whereas 29.0% of women who lived in households at least 350% above the poverty level were obese [18].

Finally, the CDC found that the prevalence of obesity increased in adults at all income and education levels between 1988 and 2008. In other words, an important finding was made that most adults with obesity were not low income [19].

Global prevalence of obesity in adults

The increase in the prevalence of obesity is replicated across affluent countries as well. All countries witnessed an increase in the prevalence of obesity of at least 22% between 2000 and 2015 (Fig. 7 and Table 8). Israel had the lowest percentage increase in prevalence of 22.3%, from 21.1% in 2000 to 25.8% in 2015. Japan had the highest percentage increase of 95.2%, from 2.1% in 2000 to 4.1% in 2015. Ireland had the second highest percentage increase of 54.4%, from 16% in 2000 to 24.7% in 2015.

Similar to the United States, the distribution of the prevalence of obesity is heterogeneous. Relative and absolute inequalities by occupation were observed in all countries [20]. Societies with a low degree of inequality (such as Japan or Scandinavian countries with narrow income differences) seem to have a lower obesity burden then more unequal societies (the United Kingdom and Australia).

Globally, stark regional differences exist across all WHO regions (Table 9). In 2016, the prevalence of obesity among adults was lowest in Southeast Asia and the Western Pacific at 4.7% and 6.4%, respectively. The prevalence was highest in the Americas at 28.6%. Europe followed with a prevalence of 23.5%, then the Eastern Mediterranean at 20.8%, and finally Africa at 10.8%.

When divided by sex, women had a higher prevalence in comparison to men in every region. The difference was largest in the Eastern Mediterranean and Africa, where the prevalence of obesity among women was 10.3% and 9.7%,

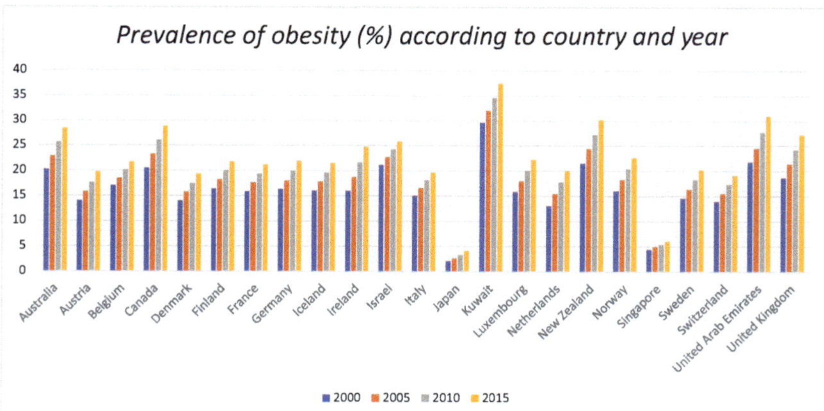

FIG. 7 Trend of obesity prevalence among affluent countries. All countries observed an increase in prevalence from 2000 to 2015. *Adapted from WHO, Global Health Observatory.*

TABLE 8 Trend of obesity (%) according to country and year from 2000 to 2015.

	2000	2005	2010	2015
Australia	20.2	22.9	25.6	28.4
Austria	14.0	15.8	17.6	19.7
Belgium	17.0	18.5	20.1	21.7
Canada	20.5	23.3	26.0	28.8
Denmark	14.0	15.7	17.4	19.3
Finland	16.4	18.2	20.0	21.8
France	15.8	17.6	19.3	21.2
Germany	16.3	18.0	19.9	21.9
Iceland	16.0	17.8	19.6	21.5
Ireland	16.0	18.7	21.6	24.7
Israel	21.1	22.7	24.2	25.8
Italy	15.0	16.5	18.1	19.6
Japan	2.1	2.6	3.3	4.1
Kuwait	29.6	32	34.6	37.4
Luxembourg	15.8	17.9	20.0	22.2
Netherlands	13.0	15.4	17.7	20
New Zealand	21.5	24.4	27.2	30.2
Norway	16.0	18.2	20.4	22.6
Qatar	4.4	4.9	5.4	6
Singapore	14.6	16.3	18.2	20.2
Sweden	13.9	15.5	17.3	19.1
Switzerland	21.8	24.5	27.7	31
United Arab Emirates	18.6	21.4	24.2	27.2
United Kingdom	20.2	22.9	25.6	28.4

Adapted from WHO, Global Health Observatory—body mass index (BMI); prevalence of obesity among adults, BMI $\geq$30, age-standardized; estimates by country; year 2000–2015.

TABLE 9 **Prevalence of obesity among adults: 2016 estimates by WHO region.**

WHO region	Both sexes (%)	Male (%)	Female (%)
Africa	10.6	5.6	15.3
Americas	28.6	25.9	31.0
Southeast Asia	4.7	3.3	6.1
Europe	23.3	21.9	24.5
Eastern Mediterranean	20.8	15.7	26.0
Western Pacific	6.4	6.0	6.7

Adapted from WHO, Global Health Observatory—body mass index (BMI); prevalence of obesity among adults, BMI $\geq$30, age-standardized; estimates by WHO region; year 2016.

TABLE 10 **Prevalence of obesity among adults: 2016 estimates by World Bank income group.**

World Bank income group	Both sexes (%)	Male (%)	Female (%)
Low income	6.8	3.6	9.9
Lower middle income	7.6	5.3	9.9
Upper middle income	13.8	11.3	16.2
High income	24.6	24.5	24.7

Adapted from WHO, Global Health Observatory—body mass index (BMI); prevalence of obesity among adults, BMI $\geq$30, age-standardized; estimates by World Bank income group; year 2016.

respectively, higher than men. The difference was smallest in the Western Pacific at 0.7% between females and males.

The disparity of obesity prevalence between men and women persists even when stratified according to World Bank income groups (Table 10). The size of the difference between men and women was negatively correlated with the income group. However, the prevalence of obesity for both sexes was positively correlated with the income group.

Prevalence of obesity in children and adolescents

The prevalence of childhood obesity (2–19 years) has a positive linear trend similar to that of adults (Fig. 8 and Table 11). In 2016, the prevalence of

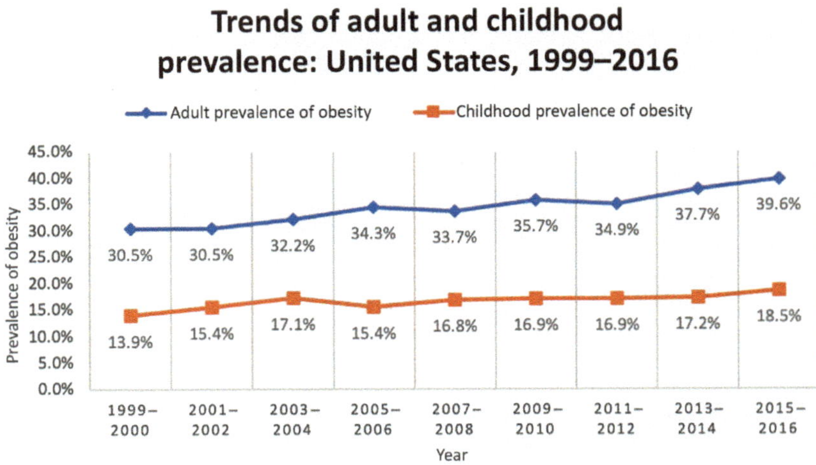

FIG. 8 Trends of adult and childhood obesity prevalence in the United States. Both age brackets observed an increase in prevalence from 1999 to 2016. *Adapted from NCHS Data Brief, no. 288, Oct. 2017.*

TABLE 11 Trends of adult and childhood prevalence: United States, 1999–2016.

Year	Adult prevalence of obesity (%)	Childhood prevalence of obesity (%)
1999–2000	30.5	13.9
2001–2002	30.5	15.4
2003–2004	32.2	17.1
2005–2006	34.3	15.4
2007–2008	33.7	16.8
2009–10	35.7	16.9
2011–12	34.9	16.9
2013–14	37.7	17.2
2015–16	39.6	18.5

Adapted from NCHS Data Brief, no. 288, Oct. 2017.

TABLE 12 Prevalence of obesity among youth aged 2–19 years: United States, 2015–16.

Age	Boys (%)	Girls (%)
2–5 years	14.3	13.5
6–11 years	20.4	16.3
12–19 years	20.2	20.9

Adapted from NCHS Data Brief, no. 288, Oct. 2017.

childhood obesity was 18.5% with 5.6% with severe obesity and 16.6% as overweight. Adolescents (12–19 years) had the highest prevalence at 20.6%, followed by school-aged children (6–11 years) at 18.4% and preschool-aged children (2–5 years) at 13.9% [5]. There was no significant difference in the prevalence of obesity between girls and boys [5]. Interestingly, the rate of increase in prevalence over childhood was different between girls and boys (Table 12). The greatest increase in prevalence for boys occurred between preschool age and school age (14.3% and 20.4%), whereas for girls this occurred between school age and adolescence (16.3% and 20.9%) [5].

The prevalence of obesity among non-Hispanic African Americans (22.0%) and Hispanic youth (25.8%) was higher than among both non-Hispanic white (14.1%) and non-Hispanic Asian (11.0%) youth [5]. The pattern among girls was similar to the pattern in all youth. The pattern among boys was similar to the pattern in all youth, except Hispanic boys had a higher prevalence of obesity than non-Hispanic African American boys [5].

In other affluent countries, obesity has markedly risen in children and adolescents over the last two decades, even though noticeable variations in the estimations across countries have been reported (Tables 13 and 14). The Netherlands had the highest percent increase in the prevalence of obesity among children age 5–9 of 69.8%, from 5.3% in 2000 to 9% in 2015. Belgium had the lowest percent increase in the prevalence of obesity among children of 4.9%, from 8.2% in 2000 to 8.6% in 2015. This pattern was replicated among adolescents age 10–19: The Netherlands had the largest percent increase of 88.4% (from 3.2% in 2000 to 5.9% in 2015) and Belgium the lowest of 5.3% (from 5.7% in 2000 to 6.0% in 2015).

Future trends

The projections of future trends worldwide are grim. By 2025, the global obesity prevalence is expected to reach 18% in men and surpass 21% in women; severe obesity will surpass 6% in men and 9% in women [21]. Forecasts based

TABLE 13 Crude estimates of prevalence of obesity (%) among children age 5–9, according to country and year.

	2000	2005	2010	2015
Australia	11.1	12.6	13.5	14.3
Austria	7.1	8.1	9.1	10.2
Belgium	8.2	8.4	8.5	8.6
Canada	10.1	11.7	12.9	14.0
Denmark	8.5	8.8	9.0	9.2
Finland	9.0	9.9	10.7	11.6
France	7.4	8.3	9.2	10.1
Germany	8.4	9.3	10.2	11.2
Iceland	10.8	11.4	11.9	12.5
Ireland	7.6	9.3	10.7	12.2
Israel	12.8	13.6	14.2	14.7
Italy	13.9	15.3	16.5	17.6
Japan	4.5	4.8	5.0	5.1
Kuwait	17.8	19.7	21.4	22.8
Luxembourg	8.5	9.4	10.2	11.0
Netherlands	5.3	6.5	7.8	9.0
Norway	7.9	8.9	9.9	10.8
Qatar	16.6	18.7	20.7	22.5
Singapore	8.5	8.8	9.1	9.4
Sweden	6.3	6.9	7.4	8.1
Switzerland	5.1	5.6	6.2	7.0
United Arab Emirates	12.9	15.4	17.8	20.0
United Kingdom	9.6	10.8	11.3	11.5

Adapted from WHO, Global Health Observatory—body mass index (BMI); prevalence of obesity among children and adolescents; year 2000–2015.

on the linear time trend suggest that 51% of the US population will be obese by 2030. Current trends place countries in Europe on a trajectory similar to the United States regarding obesity. However, because of the inherent difficulties with the calculation of accurate predictions of the future, a moderate amount of uncertainty remains with current projections.

TABLE 14 **Crude estimates of prevalence of obesity (%) among children age 10–19, according to country and year.**

Country	2000	2005	2010	2015
Australia	8.5	9.7	10.4	11.1
Austria	5.1	5.9	6.6	7.6
Belgium	5.7	5.9	5.8	6.0
Canada	7.9	9.2	10.2	11.2
Denmark	5.6	5.9	5.9	6.1
Finland	5.7	6.4	6.8	7.6
France	4.8	5.4	6.1	6.8
Germany	5.5	6.1	6.8	7.6
Iceland	7.0	7.5	7.8	8.3
Ireland	4.5	5.7	6.9	8.0
Israel	8.5	9.1	9.6	10.1
Italy	7.1	8.1	8.8	9.7
Japan	2.2	2.4	2.5	2.5
Kuwait	17.6	19.5	21.1	22.5
Luxembourg	5.2	5.8	6.3	6.9
Netherlands	3.2	4.1	5.0	5.9
New Zealand	10.2	11.9	13.2	14.7
Norway	5.6	6.4	7.1	7.9
Qatar	12.0	14.0	15.6	17.3
Singapore	5.2	5.3	5.4	5.6
Sweden	4.3	4.7	5.0	5.7
Switzerland	3.6	4.0	4.4	5.0
United Arab Emirates	8.7	10.4	11.7	14.2
United Kingdom	7.9	8.9	9.3	9.4

Adapted from WHO, Global Health Observatory—body mass index (BMI); prevalence of obesity among children and adolescents; estimates by country; year 2000–2015.

References

[1] GBD 2015 Obesity Collaborators. Afshin A, Forouzanfar MH, et al. Health effects of overweight and obesity in 195 countries over 25 years. N Engl J Med 2017;377(1):13–27. https://doi.org/10.1056/NEJMoa1614362.

[2] Stevens GA, Singh GM, Lu Y, et al. National, regional, and global trends in adult overweight and obesity prevalences. Popul Health Metr 2012;10:22. https://doi.org/10.1186/1478-7954-10-22.

[3] Blüher M. Obesity: global epidemiology and pathogenesis. Nat Rev Endocrinol 2019;15(5):288–98. https://doi.org/10.1038/s41574-019-0176-8.

[4] Gender Statistics | DataBank. https://databank.worldbank.org/reports.aspx?source=283and series=SH.STA.OB18.MA.ZS. [Accessed 27 February 2020].

[5] Hales CM, Carroll MD, Fryar CD, Ogden CL. Prevalence of obesity among adults and youth: United States, 2015–2016, NCHS Data Brief 2017;(288):1–8. https://pubmed.ncbi.nlm.nih.gov/29155689.

[6] GNI per capita, Atlas method (current US$) | Data. https://data.worldbank.org/indicator/NY.GNP.PCAP.CD?view=chart. [Accessed 29 February 2020].

[7] Purnell JQ. Definitions, classification, and epidemiology of obesity, MDText.com; 2018. http://www.ncbi.nlm.nih.gov/pubmed/25905390. [Accessed 8 March 2020].

[8] Executive summary. Obes Res 1998;6(S2):51S–179S. https://doi.org/10.1002/j.1550-8528.1998.tb00690.x.

[9] Hales CM, Carroll MD, Fryar CDOC. Prevalence of obesity and severe obesity among adults: United States, 2017–2018, NCHS Data Brief 2020;(360), https://www.cdc.gov/nchs/data/databriefs/db360-h.pdf.

[10] Early release of selected estimates based on data from the January–June 2001 National Health Interview Survey. https://www.cdc.gov/nchs/nhis/erkeyindicators.htm. [Accessed 23 February, 2020].

[11] Vital Statistics of New York State 2001 Tables. https://www.health.ny.gov/statistics/vital_statistics/2001/toc.htm. [Accessed 23 February 2020].

[12] US Census Bureau. Statistical Abstract of the United States: 2001.

[13] Myers CA, Slack T, Martin CK, Broyles ST, Heymsfield SB. Regional disparities in obesity prevalence in the United States: a spatial regime analysis. Obesity (Silver Spring) 2015;23(2):481–7. https://doi.org/10.1002/oby.20963.

[14] Slack T, Myers CA, Martin CK, Heymsfield SB. The geographic concentration of us adult obesity prevalence and associated social, economic, and environmental factors. Obesity 2014;22(3):868–74. https://doi.org/10.1002/oby.20502.

[15] Gurka MJ, Filipp SL, Deboer MD. Geographical variation in the prevalence of obesity, metabolic syndrome, and diabetes among US adults article. Nutr Diabetes 2018;8(1) https://doi.org/10.1038/s41387-018-0024-2.

[16] Scheinker D, Valencia A, Rodriguez F. Identification of factors associated with variation in US county-level obesity prevalence rates using epidemiologic vs machine learning models. JAMA Netw Open 2019;2(4):e192884. https://doi.org/10.1001/jamanetworkopen.2019.2884.

[17] Adult Obesity Prevalence Maps | Overweight and Obesity | CDC. https://www.cdc.gov/obesity/data/prevalence-maps.html. [Accessed 24 February, 2020].

[18] Products—Data Briefs—Number 50—December 2010. https://www.cdc.gov/nchs/products/databriefs/db50.htm. [Accessed 1 March 2020].

[19] Ogden CL, Lamb MM, Carroll MD, Flegal KM. Obesity and socioeconomic status in adults: United States, 2005–2008, NCHS Data Brief 2010;(50):1–8. https://pubmed.ncbi.nlm.nih.gov/21211165.

[20] Hoffmann K, De Gelder R, Hu Y, et al. Trends in educational inequalities in obesity in 15 European countries between 1990 and 2010. Int J Behav Nutr Phys Act 2017;14(1):1–10. https://doi.org/10.1186/s12966-017-0517-8.

[21] Di Cesare M, Bentham J, Stevens GA, et al. Trends in adult body-mass index in 200 countries from 1975 to 2014: a pooled analysis of 1698 population-based measurement studies with 19.2 million participants. Lancet 2016;387(10026):1377–96. https://doi.org/10.1016/S0140-6736(16)30054-X.

Chapter 4

Etiology of obesity

Raman Mehrzad, M.D., M.H.L., M.B.A.
Department of Plastic and Reconstructive Surgery, Rhode Island Hospital, The Warren Alpert Medical School of Brown University, Providence, RI, United States

Introduction

Obesity is a chronic disease and an increasing problem globally. The prevalence is increasing in all ages—children, adolescents, and adults—and is now considered an epidemic. Obesity affects almost all physiological functions of the body and has major health consequences including, but not limited to, mental health, cancer, cardiovascular disorders, and musculoskeletal disorders [1]. All the above have negative effects on the individual, the economy, the quality of life, and work productivity.

Onset and etiology of obesity

Weight gain can occur at any age. There are obesity trends in children, adolescents, and adults. However, there are certain trends that are more common for weight gain to happen, and these also vary between genders [2]. Critical periods during the development phase are an example of times in which nutritional and environmental factors can have significant effects on the risk of becoming obese later in life. Body weight during pregnancy may predispose the mother to a larger body size and shape; it could also later influence the infant's weight and body composition [3]. Elevated body mass index (BMI), high gestational weight gain in pregnant women, and mothers with type 2 diabetes mellitus are other risk factors for childhood obesity and obesity later on in adulthood [4, 5]. Smoking during pregnancy is an additional factor for obesity [6]. Interestingly, short and small infants have been shown to raise the risk of increased abdominal circumference and obesity in adulthood [7].

Childhood and adolescence

Studies show that a significant number of obesity in adolescence is established before 5 years of age. Obesity during childhood typically also persists into adulthood. This is truer for those with a parent that is obese. Moreover, the data

Obesity. https://doi.org/10.1016/B978-0-12-818839-2.00004-1

demonstrate that there is an association between patients with obesity in adolescence and severe obesity in adulthood [7, 8]. Importantly, health events in adulthood are related to weight status in adolescence. Thus, if someone is obese at a younger age, there is a higher risk of adverse health events such as type 2 diabetes mellitus [9, 10].

Females

After the onset of puberty is when most women become overweight [11]. There is a relationship between higher adult BMI and earlier onset of puberty [12], although this weight gain may be triggered by various factors such as menopause or pregnancy.

Pregnancy

Gaining weight during pregnancy is common. This is mostly due to the growing baby and extra fluid in the body, which is needed for the baby's circulation, amniotic fluid, and placenta. The actual weight gain varies depending on race, ethnic background, genetics, and environmental factors. However, women see a modest increase in their weight with higher central fat after the first pregnancy [13, 14].

- For women who are underweight before pregnancy (BMI of <18.5), a weight gain of 28 and 40 lb during pregnancy is normal.
- For women who are of normal weight before pregnancy (BMI of between 18.5 and 24.9), a weight gain of 25 and 35 lb during pregnancy is normal.
- For women who are overweight before pregnancy (BMI of between 25 and 29.9), a weight gain of 15 and 25 lb during pregnancy is normal.
- For women who are obese before pregnancy (BMI >30), a weight gain of 11 and 20 lb during pregnancy is normal [15].

It is important to know that once the weight gain exceeds the above BMI levels, it increases the risk of postpartum weight retention [15].

Oral contraceptives

Studies show that most oral contraceptives do not cause significant weight gain. However, interestingly, women often complain of weight gain after taking oral contraceptives [6].

Menopause

As women age and hit menopause, their fat distribution changes relatively early [16]. Both ovarian aging as well as aging in general are associated with an increase in weight and body composition changes during menopause. According to one study, the average weight gain seen cumulatively in a 6-year period was 2.9 kg and the average circumference increase was 5.7 cm [17]. The same study showed that 1 year after the final menstrual period, the fat mass continued to increase, although the rate of increase in waist circumference slowed [17]. Although estrogen therapy may decrease fat redistribution, it does not help in preventing weight gain in postmenopausal women [18, 19]. Another substudy with a 3-year follow up demonstrated that women lost significantly less lean soft tissue mass when taking estrogen and progesterone therapy compared to a placebo (−0.04 vs −0.44 kg) [18]. The ratio of trunk-to-leg fat mass was also less in the intervention group; however, these effects were small and it is not clear whether these changes have significant health benefits [18, 19].

Male

Men see an increase in body weight until the sixth decade. However, after ages 55–64, weight gain remains largely stable and then in fact begins to decline [6]. There is an association of weight gain in men if they transition from an active lifestyle during their teens and twenties to a more sedentary lifestyle thereafter [6]. A decrease in serum testosterone levels in men is associated with a decrease in muscle mass and an increase in fat mass in older men [6].

Built-in environment

Numerous studies have shown an association between uncontrolled expansion of urban areas (urban sprawl) and obesity. Low-density land uses, decentralization, and automobile-focused transportation systems have all been associated with obesity [20–23]. Two studies attempted to examine the obesity relationships with community design, physical activity, and time spent in cars in Atlanta, GA, and Seattle/King County, WA. They found an association between the number of intersections, the size of blocks, the ability to get from one part of a location to another in a direct manner or through multiple pathways, physical activity, and obesity [24, 25]. Another study found that residents were more likely to walk if the neighborhoods were built before 1973. This was hypothesized by the authors to be secondary to walkable destinations, highly connected street patterns, and other amenities that might affect the obesity risk [26]. Moreover, sidewalks, accessible parks, the presence of public transportation, and other built-in environmental factors have been demonstrated in other studies to affect rates of physical activity and thereby the obesity risk [27–30].

Access to food

The obesity risk may also be due to the presence of supermarkets in different locations. Accessibility to high-quality and affordable food is related to better diet and nutrition, research suggests [31], and these types of food are less likely to be found in convenience stores but more likely to be found in supermarkets. People who prepare meals at home, presumably with ingredients bought at supermarkets, rather than those who purchase premade meals at a take-out restaurant are less likely to become obese [32]. Tactlessly, in nonwhite and low-income neighborhoods, evidence shows that supermarkets are less frequently found [23].

Lifetime

A prospective cohort study of 4117 normal-weight men and women of ages 30–59 showed that at the baseline, within 4 years 26–30% of men and 14–19% of women became overweight while 5–9% became obese. Within 30 years, the same study demonstrated that more than 50% of the study participants became overweight; 25% and 30% of the men and women, respectively, became obese [33]. Most of the participants in this study were Caucasian and of normal weight. Thus, the overall long-term risk of becoming obese or overweight over the course of an individual's life seems to be high.

Behavioral factors

It is not surprising that a sedentary lifestyle results in weight gain. This is caused by lower energy expenditure, which expedites age-related loss in lean mass and thereby causes weight gain. There are many studies that have proven this. One paper analyzed occupational activity in America over the past 50 years and found that energy-sparing devices, such as people working with computers in their workplace or at home, reduced the expenditure of energy and was associated with an increase in weight [34]. The National Health and Nutrition Examination Survey (NHANES) showed that moderate vigorous physical activity was inversely related to obesity while sedentary time or television time was positively related to obesity [35]. The Surgeon General's Report of Physical Activity demonstrated that as age increase, the percentage of adult American's involving themselves in physical activity decreases steadily. The same study showed that lower energy expenditure in children and adults predicts weight gain [36]. Prolonged television watching seem to be the highest predictive behavior of obesity and diabetes risk of all sedentary behaviors [36]. A 23% (95% CI 17–30%) increase in the risk of obesity and a 14% (95% CI 5–23%) increase in the risk of diabetes were demonstrated in the Nurses' Health Study for every 2 h spent watching TV. This was after adjusting for exercise level, age, smoking, and dietary factors [37]. The consequences of watching TV are mainly secondary to changes in energy intake rather than the physical activity alone associated with it [38, 39]. Sitting during work time and other sedentary behaviors were less associated with a risk of obesity.

Disabilities

In adults with mental health, sensory, or physical disabilities, there is a higher prevalence of obesity [40].

Diet

Diet and the risk of obesity will be discussed separately. However, poor diet has a strong relation to obesity and the changes in global food supply may be a big part of the rising prevalence of obesity [41]. The quantity of fat and refined carbohydrates has increased in the United States since 1970 and this has in turn resulted in a higher calorie intake. The biggest components that have contributed to a rise in obesity, not only in the United States but also worldwide, are portion sizes for prepared food, increasing trends in the glycemic index of foods, school nutrition content, and the increased amounts of fast food service and sugar-containing beverages. This combined with a decline in overall physical activity has meaningfully increased the burden of the obesity trend [41].

In general, dies high in sugars and fats are associated with obesity. Everything from sugar beverages, potato chips, unprocessed red meat, and processed meat have been demonstrated in epidemiological data to be directly associated with weight gain [42] while yogurt, fruits, nuts, whole grains, and vegetables are inversely associated with weight gain. Sugary beverages are a big issue in the United States. Nearly every fast food chain and outdoor dining location offers sugary beverages, and they are often included in meals that are for purchase. Moreover, many chains offer free refills, which in turn increases the calorie intake further. There is now evidence that the consumption of these sugary beverages, including fruit juice, is directly linked to the development of obesity in some individuals [43]. Genetic data show that adults who consume high intakes of sugary beverages and also have a higher genetic predisposition score have a higher association with increased adiposity [44, 45].

The microbiome has been a big research topic over the past few years and we now know that different gut floras could have various effects on the fat metabolism. Sweeteners, high processed foods, and other artificial additives could possibly impact individual weight outside the scope of calories through changes in the microbiome, either directly or indirectly [46]. This area is of major interest and there are many trials ongoing with no definitive results currently that would change recommendations.

Eating patterns play an important role in obesity as well. Most obese people have lost control of their eating patterns. Overeating relative to the loss of energy will logically cause obesity [47]. While overeating has been studied to cause obesity, the frequency of the amount of meals per day is still unclear. There are studies that show that multiple meals per day are associated with a lower risk of obesity [48, 49]. However, this is largely dependent on the amount of calories that are consumed per day, and this is also the key factor to weight change in general. The difference in insulin secretion associated with a few large meals versus small frequent meals could be one of the factors to less obesity risk with the latter [50]. Large meals result in more insulin secretion than small meals.

Another risk factor for obesity is night-eating syndrome, which is defined as eating at least 25% of the daily energy consumption at night [51]. This behavior is seen among obese people. The binge-eating disorder is another risk factor for weight gain. These people have uncontrolled episodes of eating, typically during night [51]. This is a psychiatric illness and could respond to certain antidepressive therapies.

Poor sleeping behaviors are also associated with obesity. Data show an increased trend of adult Americans who sleep less than 7h a night, which is now the recommended minimum sleep amount (changed from the 6h minimum) by the American Sleep Association [52]. Over the past 40 years, the number of adults who sleep less than 7h has increased from 16% to 37% [53]. Data show that poor sleep or sleep deprivation results in negative metabolic changes [54]. When subjects were randomized to undergo either sleep extension (10h per night) or sleep restriction (4h per night) during a 6-week period with controlled calorie intake and physical activity conditions, sleep restriction was associated with an increase in serum ghrelin (an orexigenic hormone), and increased hunger and appetite (especially for high-calorie foods and high carbohydrate content) and a decrease in serum leptin (an anorexigenic hormone) [55]. Other observational studies demonstrated similar findings with an association between sleep restriction and obesity [56, 57] as well as lowering the chances of weight loss when sleep deprived [58].

Data suggest that a calorie restrictive diet, at least for a few hours per day, could be beneficial for weight loss [58].

Smoking

Many people complain of weight gain after they stop smoking. This is, in fact, a common concern of those who want to quit smoking. The weight gain seen in smoking cessation is mediated by an increase in food intake and less physical activity as a result of nicotine withdrawal [59]. However, the increase in weight is on average 4–5kg over a few months, although it could be greater [59, 60]. There is an increase in the odds ratio of obesity with smoking cessation compared to nonsmokers by 2 in women and 2.4 in men. Exercise programs and a low-calorie diet are recommended to prevent the weight gain associated with smoking cessation [61].

Medical conditions

Many medical conditions can lead to obesity by altering the body weight. Some of the typical examples are polycystic ovary syndrome, Cushing's syndrome, hypothyroidism, and growth hormone deficiency. In Cushing's syndrome, an excess in glucocorticoids is seen that induces 11-beta-hydroxysteroid dehydrogenase type 1 in visceral fat, which in turn results in increased lipogenic capacity in visceral fat [62]. In hypothyroidism, there is a decrease in metabolism that causes a modest weight gain [63, 64]. Thus, different hormonal activities alter the metabolism, which leads to an increase in weight in the population. Some of these situations are not yet not fully understood, such as in polycystic ovary syndrome.

Mental health

Mental disorders could lead to obesity. Psychological aspects are important when it comes to eating behaviors, physical activity, a sedentary lifestyle, and other factors that contribute to calorie excess. One of the cardinal symptoms in depression is weight change, either weight gain or loss. While some people eat less, others tend to eat more when depressed [65]. Similarly, seasonal depressive disorder is a condition where people feel symptoms of depression during winter, and this condition has been linked to weight gain. People with attention-deficit hyperactivity disorder (ADHD) also have a higher risk of obesity [66].

Various medications that treat psychiatric disorders have effects on weight gain. Antidepressants are a group of medications for the treatment of depression. Imipramine, amitriptyline, clomipramine, and doxepin are tricyclic antidepressants that are associated with weight gain. The long-term use of some selective serotonin reuptake inhibitors (SSRIs) has been demonstrated in a study to cause weight gain [67]. Antipsychotics can have different effects on weight. For instance, first-generation antipsychotics such as thioridazine caused the highest weight gain, roughly 3.2kg after 10weeks. Risperidone, clozapine, and olanzapine are examples of second-generation antipsychotics associated with the greatest weight gain with 2.1kg, 4.4kg, and 4.2kg, respectively [68]. Lithium is another medication for mental health disorders that is a mood stabilizer in bipolar disorder and is associated with weight gain.

Medications

In general, many prescription medications can cause weight gain. The exact effect of the weight gain varies depending on the medication, but overall the mechanism can be through different approaches such as slowed metabolism, fluid retention, increased appetite, increased fat storage, and/or impaired exercise tolerance (Table 1).

Insulin therapy for diabetes cause changes in weight gain. In the Diabetes Control and Complications Trial, a 5.1kg weight gain was seen in the intensive-treatment group [69]. Antidiabetic medications such as sulfonylureas, rosiglitazone, thiazolidinediones, and pioglitazone are all associated with

TABLE 1 Medications that alter weight in patients.

Produce weight gain	Produce weight loss	Are weight neutral
Antidepressants: monoamine oxidase inhibitors, tricyclic antidepressants (nortriptyline, amitriptyline, doxepin), paroxetine, citalopram, escitalopram, imipramine, mirtazapine	Anticonvulsants: topiramate, zonisamide, lamotrigine	Antipsychotics: haloperidol, aripiprazole
Antipsychotics: thioridazine, olanzapine, risperidone, clozapine, quetiapine	Antidepressants: bupropion, venlafaxine, desvenlafaxine	
Diabetes medications: e.g., insulin, sulfonylureas, thiazolidinediones, meglitinides	Antipsychotics: ziprasidone	
Glucocorticoids: e.g., prednisone		
Hormonal agents: especially progestins, e.g., medroxyprogesterone		
Anticonvulsants: e.g., divalproex		
Neurologic and mood-stabilizing agents: e.g., lithium, carbamazepine, gabapentin, valproate		
Antihistamines: cyproheptadine		
Alpha blockers: especially terazosin		
Beta blockers: especially propranolol Opioids		

weight gain [68]. There are, however, medications in the same class that cause weight loss. A few examples of these are metformin, glucagon-like peptide-1 [GLP-1] receptor agonists, sodium-glucose co-transporter 2 [SGLT2] inhibitors, alpha-glucosidase inhibitors [6, 70].

Carbamazepine and valproate acid are examples of antiepileptics that are used in both epilepsy and bipolar disorder. Both these drugs cause weight gain [6].

Beta blockers, glucocorticoid, and cyproheptadine (antihistamine) all cause weight gain [68]. Opioids such as oxycodone may decrease the metabolism and exercise tolerance, which could lead to weight gain [7].

Consequently, patients who receive any of the above medications should be aware of the potential side effect on their weight and these patients should be assisted in finding strategies to maintain their weight if these medications are required to be taken.

Socioeconomic factors

In general, lower socioeconomic groups have a higher prevalence of obesity [71]. The causes of this are multifactorial and not entirely clear. However, financial status, food environments, elements of the built environment, all-round education, and nutritional education are likely related to this [72, 73].

Ethnicity

There seems to be a relation between obesity and ethnic background as well. Black women of all ages are more obese than white women while black men are less obese than white men. White women and men have a higher prevalence of obesity than white men and women [74]. Interestingly, obesity onset in young adulthood is faster in hispanic and black women compared to white women [75]. Other studies have found that the racial individualities of districts do influence obesity risk [76, 77].

References

[1] Chooi YC, Ding C, Magkos F. The epidemiology of obesity. Metabolism 2019 Mar;92:6–10. https://doi.org/10.1016/j.metabol.2018.09.005.

[2] Ozanne SE. Epigenetic signatures of obesity. N Engl J Med 2015;372:973.

[3] Oken E, Taveras EM, Kleinman KP, et al. Gestational weight gain and child adiposity at age 3 years. Am J Obstet Gynecol 2007;196:322.e1.

[4] Bray GA. A guide to obesity and the metabolic syndrome. Boca Raton, FL: CRC Press; 2011.

[5] Oken E, Levitan EB, Gillman MW. Maternal smoking during pregnancy and child overweight: systematic review and meta-analysis. Int J Obes (Lond) 2008;32:201.

[6] Perreault L, Pi-Sunyer X, Kunis L. Obesity in adults: etiology and risk factors. UpToDate; Oct 2018. Available at: https://www.uptodate.com/contents/obesity-in-adults-etiology-and-risk-factors?search=etiology%20of%20obesity&source=search_result&selectedTitle=1~150&usage_type=default&display_rank=1.

[7] Loos RJ. Genetic determinants of common obesity and their value in prediction. Best Pract Res Clin Endocrinol Metab 2012;26:211.

[8] The NS, Suchindran C, North KE, et al. Association of adolescent obesity with risk of severe obesity in adulthood. JAMA 2010;304:2042.

[9] Must A, Phillips SM, Naumova EN. Occurrence and timing of childhood overweight and mortality: findings from the Third Harvard Growth Study. J Pediatr 2012;160:743.

[10] Bjerregaard LG, Jensen BW, Ängquist L, et al. Change in overweight from childhood to early adulthood and risk of type 2 diabetes. N Engl J Med 2018;378:1302.

[11] Deshmukh-Taskar P, Nicklas TA, Morales M, et al. Tracking of overweight status from childhood to young adulthood: the Bogalusa Heart Study. Eur J Clin Nutr 2006;60:48.

[12] Gill D, Brewer CF, Del Greco MF, et al. Age at menarche and adult body mass index: a Mendelian randomization study. Int J Obes (Lond) 2018;42:1574.

[13] Smith DE, Lewis CE, Caveny JL, et al. Longitudinal changes in adiposity associated with pregnancy. The CARDIA Study Coronary Artery Risk Development in Young Adults Study. JAMA 1994;271:1747.

[14] Gunderson EP, Sternfeld B, Wellons MF, et al. Childbearing may increase visceral adipose tissue independent of overall increase in body fat. Obesity (Silver Spring) 2008;16:1078.

[15] https://www.ncbi.nlm.nih.gov/books/NBK279575/.
[16] Lovejoy JC. The menopause and obesity. Prim Care 2003;30:317.
[17] Sowers M, Zheng H, Tomey K, et al. Changes in body composition in women over six years at midlife: ovarian and chronological aging. J Clin Endocrinol Metab 2007;92:895.
[18] Chen Z, Bassford T, Green SB, et al. Postmenopausal hormone therapy and body composition—a substudy of the estrogen plus progestin trial of the Women's Health Initiative. Am J Clin Nutr 2005;82:651.
[19] Espeland MA, Stefanick ML, Kritz-Silverstein D, et al. Effect of postmenopausal hormone therapy on body weight and waist and hip girths. Postmenopausal Estrogen-Progestin Interventions Study Investigators. J Clin Endocrinol Metab 1997;82:1549.
[20] Lopez R. Urban sprawl and risk for being overweight or obese. Am J Public Health 2004;94:1574–9.
[21] Ewing R, Schmid T, Killingsworth R, Zlot A, Raudenbush S. Relationship between urban sprawl and physical activity, obesity, and morbidity. Am J Health Promot 2003;18:47–57.
[22] Sturm R, Cohen D. Suburban sprawl and physical and mental health. Public Health 2004;118:488–96.
[23] Morland K, Wing S, Diez-Roux A, Poole C. Neighborhood characteristics associated with the location of food stores and food service places. Am J Prev Med 2001;22:23–9.
[24] Frank L, Andersen M, Schmid T. Obesity relationships with community design, physical activity, and time spent in cars. Am J Prev Med 2004;27:87–96.
[25] Frank L, Sallis J, Conway T, Chapman J, Saelens B, Bachman W. Many pathways from land use to health. J Am Plann Assoc 2006;72:75–87.
[26] Berrigan D, Troiano R. The association between urban form and physical activity in U.S. adults. Am J Prev Med 2002;23(Suppl. 2):74–9.
[27] Sallis J, Rochaska J, Taylor W. A review of correlates of physical activity of children and adolescents. Med Sci Sports Exerc 2000;32:963–75.
[28] Ross C. Walking, exercising, and smoking: does neighborhood matter? Soc Sci Med 2000;51:265–74.
[29] Saelens B, Sallis J, Black J, Chen D. Neighborhood-based differences in physical activity: an environmental scale evaluation. Am J Public Health 2003;93:1552–8.
[30] King W, Brach J, Belle S, Killingsworth R, Fenton M, Kriska A. The relationship between convenience of destinations and walking levels in older women. Am J Health Promot 2003;18:74–82.
[31] Morland K, Wing S, Diez-Roux A. The contextual effect of the local food environment on residents'diets: the atherosclerosis risk in communities study. Am J Public Health 2002;92:1761–7.
[32] McCrory M, Suen V, Roberts S. Biobehavioral influences on energy intake and adult weight gain. J Nutr 2002;132(Suppl):3830–4.
[33] Vasan RS, Pencina MJ, Cobain M, et al. Estimated risks for developing obesity in the Framingham Heart Study. Ann Intern Med 2005;143:473.
[34] Church TS, Thomas DM, Tudor-Locke C, et al. Trends over 5 decades in U.S. occupation-related physical activity and their associations with obesity. PLoS One 2011;6:e19657.
[35] Maher CA, Mire E, Harrington DM, et al. The independent and combined associations of physical activity and sedentary behavior with obesity in adults: NHANES 2003–06. Obesity (Silver Spring) 2013;21:E730.
[36] US Department of Health and Human Services. Physical activity and health: a report of the surgeon general. Atlanta, GA: US Department of Health and Human Services; 1996.
[37] Hu FB, Li TY, Colditz GA, et al. Television watching and other sedentary behaviors in relation to risk of obesity and type 2 diabetes mellitus in women. JAMA 2003;289:1785.

[38] Borghese MM, Tremblay MS, Leduc G, et al. Independent and combined associations of total sedentary time and television viewing time with food intake patterns of 9- to 11-year-old Canadian children. Appl Physiol Nutr Metab 2014;39:937.
[39] Bellisle F. Meals and snacking, diet quality and energy balance. Physiol Behav 2014;134:38.
[40] Weil E, Wachterman M, McCarthy EP, et al. Obesity among adults with disabling conditions. JAMA 2002;288:1265.
[41] Swinburn BA, Sacks G, Hall KD, et al. The global obesity pandemic: shaped by global drivers and local environments. Lancet 2011;378:804.
[42] Mozaffarian D, Hao T, Rimm EB, et al. Changes in diet and lifestyle and long-term weight gain in women and men. N Engl J Med 2011;364:2392.
[43] Malik VS, Pan A, Willett WC, Hu FB. Sugar-sweetened beverages and weight gain in children and adults: a systematic review and meta-analysis. Am J Clin Nutr 2013;98:1084.
[44] Qi Q, Chu AY, Kang JH, et al. Sugar-sweetened beverages and genetic risk of obesity. N Engl J Med 2012;367:1387.
[45] McCaffery JM, Papandonatos GD, Peter I, et al. Obesity susceptibility loci and dietary intake in the Look AHEAD Trial. Am J Clin Nutr 2012;95:1477.
[46] Azad MB, Abou-Setta AM, Chauhan BF, et al. Nonnutritive sweeteners and cardiometabolic health: a systematic review and meta-analysis of randomized controlled trials and prospective cohort studies. CMAJ 2017;189:E929.
[47] Bouchard C, Tremblay A, Després JP, et al. The response to long-term overfeeding in identical twins. N Engl J Med 1990;322:1477.
[48] Jääskeläinen A, Schwab U, Kolehmainen M, et al. Associations of meal frequency and breakfast with obesity and metabolic syndrome traits in adolescents of Northern Finland Birth Cohort 1986. Nutr Metab Cardiovasc Dis 2013;23:1002.
[49] Toschke AM, Thorsteinsdottir KH, von Kries R, GME Study Group. Meal frequency, breakfast consumption and childhood obesity. Int J Pediatr Obes 2009;4:242.
[50] Bhutani S, Varady KA. Nibbling versus feasting: which meal pattern is better for heart disease prevention? Nutr Rev 2009;67:591.
[51] Allison KC, Grilo CM, Masheb RM, Stunkard AJ. Binge eating disorder and night eating syndrome: a comparative study of disordered eating. J Consult Clin Psychol 2005;73:1107.
[52] Sleep Association. Available at: https://www.sleepassociation.org/blog-post/much-sleep-need/.
[53] National Sleep Foundation. Sleep in America Poll. Washington, DC: National Sleep Foundation; 2002.
[54] Markwald RR, Melanson EL, Smith MR, et al. Impact of insufficient sleep on total daily energy expenditure, food intake, and weight gain. Proc Natl Acad Sci U S A 2013;110:5695.
[55] Spiegel K, Tasali E, Penev P, Van Cauter E. Brief communication: sleep curtailment in healthy young men is associated with decreased leptin levels, elevated ghrelin levels, and increased hunger and appetite. Ann Intern Med 2004;141:846.
[56] Patel SR, Hu FB. Short sleep duration and weight gain: a systematic review. Obesity (Silver Spring) 2008;16:643.
[57] Cappuccio FP, Taggart FM, Kandala NB, et al. Meta-analysis of short sleep duration and obesity in children and adults. Sleep 2008;31:619.
[58] Nedeltcheva AV, Kilkus JM, Imperial J, et al. Insufficient sleep undermines dietary efforts to reduce adiposity. Ann Intern Med 2010;153:435.
[59] Filozof C, Fernández Pinilla MC, Fernández-Cruz A. Smoking cessation and weight gain. Obes Rev 2004;5:95.
[60] Leslie WS, Koshy PR, Mackenzie M, et al. Changes in body weight and food choice in those attempting smoking cessation: a cluster randomised controlled trial. BMC Public Health 2012;12:389.

[61] Parsons AC, Shraim M, Inglis J, et al. Interventions for preventing weight gain after smoking cessation. Cochrane Database Syst Rev 2009;CD006219.

[62] Morton NM, Seckl JR. 11beta-hydroxysteroid dehydrogenase type 1 and obesity. Front Horm Res 2008;36:146.

[63] Knudsen N, Laurberg P, Rasmussen LB, et al. Small differences in thyroid function may be important for body mass index and the occurrence of obesity in the population. J Clin Endocrinol Metab 2005;90:4019.

[64] Fox CS, Pencina MJ, D'Agostino RB, et al. Relations of thyroid function to body weight: cross-sectional and longitudinal observations in a community-based sample. Arch Intern Med 2008;168:587.

[65] Malhi GS, Mann JJ. Depression. Lancet 2018 Nov 24;392(10161):2299–312. https://doi.org/10.1016/S0140-6736(18)31948-2.

[66] Dickerson F, Brown C, Kreyenbuhl J, et al. Obesity among individuals with serious mental illness. Acta Psychiatr Scand 2006;113(4):6–313.

[67] Fava M, Judge R, Hoog SL, et al. Fluoxetine versus sertraline and paroxetine in major depressive disorder: changes in weight with long-term treatment. J Clin Psychiatry 2000;61:863.

[68] Leslie WS, Hankey CR, Lean ME. Weight gain as an adverse effect of some commonly prescribed drugs: a systematic review. QJM 2007;100:395.

[69] Weight gain associated with intensive therapy in the diabetes control and complications trial. The DCCT Research Group. Diabetes Care 1988;11:567.

[70] Knowler WC, Barrett-Connor E, Fowler SE, et al. Reduction in the incidence of type 2 diabetes with lifestyle intervention or metformin. N Engl J Med 2002;346:393.

[71] Drewnowski A, Rehm CD, Solet D. Disparities in obesity rates: analysis by ZIP code area. Soc Sci Med 2007;65:2458.

[72] Drewnowski A. The economics of food choice behavior: why poverty and obesity are linked. Nestle Nutr Inst Workshop Ser 2012;73:95.

[73] Dubowitz T, Ghosh-Dastidar MB, Steiner E, et al. Are our actions aligned with our evidence? The skinny on changing the landscape of obesity. Obesity (Silver Spring) 2013;21:419.

[74] Clinical guidelines on the identification, evaluation, and treatment of overweight and obesity in adults—the evidence report. National Institutes of Health. Obes Res 1998;6(Suppl. 2):51S.

[75] McTigue KM, Garrett JM, Popkin BM. The natural history of the development of obesity in a cohort of young U.S. adults between 1981 and 1998. Ann Intern Med 2002;136:857.

[76] Glass T, Rasmussen M, Schwartz B. Neighborhoods and obesity in older adults: the Baltimore memory study. Am J Prev Med 2006;31:455–63.

[77] Zhang X, Christoffel K, Mason M, Liu L. Identification of contrastive and comparable school neighborhoods for childhood obesity and physical activity research. Int J Health Geogr 2006;5:14.

Chapter 5

The global impact of obesity

Raman Mehrzad, M.D., M.H.L., M.B.A.
Department of Plastic and Reconstructive Surgery, Rhode Island Hospital, The Warren Alpert Medical School of Brown University, Providence, RI, United States

Global concerns

The global obesity epidemic is worsening around the world and unless major interventions take place, the implications will be ominous. As stated previously, the prevalence of overweight and obesity is increasing, not only in the United States but also globally [1]. Apart from tobacco, obesity is likely the biggest threat to collective health in America. Globally, it has a major health impact and the effects on individuals, communities, and nations are lasting not just today but for future generations as well.

Obesity is the second-leading cause of death of adults in the United States. Although tobacco is the number one cause, the use of tobacco is declining while the rate of obesity is continuously rising, and will soon likely exceed the death rate from tobacco use [2].

The two major concerns with obesity globally are the health and economical effects. In regard to health concerns, obesity is closely related to numerous health conditions, including but not limited to diabetes, myocardial infarction, coronary heart disease, infertility, stroke, sleep apnea, hypertension, hypercholesterolemia, asthma, and many cancers. Colon cancer, breast cancer, and leukemia are just a few cancers where obesity increases the risk. Economically, the health care cost related to obesity in the United States was $190 billion in 2005 [3]. However, although health and economical consequences are the two major concerns, there are multiple other issues that come along with obesity such as discrimination, bullying, poor quality of life, and lower wages, among other consequences [4].

An effort has been made over recent years through epidemiological studies to evaluate the trends of BMI both in the United States and in other parts of the world [5, 6] as well as to assess the effects on health outcomes [7, 8]. A study that assembled data from 195 countries showed that overweight and obesity has more than doubled since 1980 and was 12% in adults and 5% in children [1]. Although there is this increase in prevalence, the same study showed that the

Obesity. https://doi.org/10.1016/B978-0-12-818839-2.00005-3

effect of elevated BMI on death and disability has not grown, which was encouraging. This suggests that people are living longer than previously, most likely due to better health management and care. Still, people with obesity face more time with harming coexisting illnesses such as chronic kidney disease, cancers, and type 2 diabetes [1]. However, there are countries in which this may turn around. For instance, Brazil, China, and Indonesia have seen the most worrying trend with nearly a tripling rate of obesity in young adults [9]. If this continues, our medical care may not keep up to maintain the same increase in survival rate we have seen with obesity over the past few years.

Global health care concerns

Many chronic illnesses such as type 2 diabetes, chronic kidney disease, and hypertension increase in their cumulative incidences at the earlier onset of obesity. Type 2 diabetes is an example of a disease that has constantly increased in incidence in youth. Importantly, the complication rate of the disease increases the earlier the onset of the disease.

As mentioned earlier, in 2017 a study was published in the New England Journal of Medicine from the global burden of disease collaborators that examined the health effects of overweight and obesity in 195 countries over 25 years [1]. The study showed that globally among adults, overweight caused 4 million deaths and 120 million disability-adjusted life years (DALYs) in 2015. This accounted for 7.2% of all-cause deaths and 4.9% of all-cause DALYs. In 2015, the leading cause of high BMI-related deaths and DALYs was cardiovascular disease, accounting for 2.7 million deaths and 66.3 million DALYs. Diabetes was the second biggest cause of BMI-related deaths with 0.9 million deaths and 39.1 million DALYs. Chronic kidney disease was the second biggest cause of high BMI-related DALYs. Most of these consequences were in those with BMI >30 [1]. The same study showed that nearly 39% of deaths and 36% of DALYs related to high BMI occurred in those with a BMI >30 kg/m^2 [1]. Overall, cancers and chronic kidney disease contributed to <10% of all deaths while musculoskeletal disorders, diabetes, and neoplasm each accounted for <10% of all DALYs. A total of 28.6 million years lived with disability was associated with elevated BMI globally, with diabetes (19.3 million) being the leading cause followed by musculoskeletal disorders (5.7 million) [1].

Moreover, in regard to trends, the study showed an increase in global mortality related to elevated BMI by 28.3% from 1990 to 2015. However, no changes were seen in standardized mortality rates during this period. There was also an increase in DALYs by 35.8% while again no observed significant change in age-standardized rates was seen during this time [1].

Global ranks and trends in obesity

Some nations have by far a higher proportion of obese people than others. It is not the richest countries in the world have the most obese people per proportion.

Because the rising cost of healthy food is a contributing factor to obesity, many nations with smaller economies are in fact at the top [10]. In 2020, American Samoa was the most obese country in the world followed by Tokelau and Nauru. In American Samoa, 74.6% of its population has a BMI >30. Tokelau and Nauru have 74.4% and 61.0% obese people, respectively. The United States is ranked 16 (Table 1) [10].

TABLE 1 Global ranks and trends of obesity.

Country	Obesity rate	BMI	Population 2020
American Samoa	74.60%	34.9	55,191
Tokelau	74.40%		1357
Nauru	61.00%	32.5	10,824
Cook Islands	55.90%	33	17,564
Palau	55.30%	29.4	18,094
Marshall Islands	52.90%	29.2	59,190
Tuvalu	51.60%	29.3	11,792
Niue	50.00%		1626
Tonga	48.20%	31.9	105,695
Samoa	47.30%	31.7	198,414
Kiribati	46.00%	29.6	119,449
Micronesia	45.80%	29.4	115,023
Aruba	38.20%		106,766
Kuwait	37.90%	30	4,270,571
Cayman Islands	36.60%		65,722
United States	36.20%	28.8	331,002,651
British Virgin Islands	35.50%		30,231
Jordan	35.50%	28.9	10,203,134
Saudi Arabia	35.40%	28.5	34,813,871
Qatar	35.10%	29.2	2,881,053
Bermuda	34.40%		62,278
Guam	34.30%		168,775
French Polynesia	33.10%		280,908
Puerto Rico	32.90%		2,860,853

Continued

TABLE 1 Global ranks and trends of obesity—cont'd

Country	Obesity rate	BMI	Population 2020
United States Virgin Islands	32.50%		104,425
Libya	32.50%	27.7	6,871,292
Turkey	32.10%	27.8	84,339,067
Egypt	32.00%	29.2	102,334,404
Lebanon	32.00%	27.8	6,825,445
United Arab Emirates	31.70%	28.8	9,890,402
Bahamas	31.60%	28.4	393,244
New Caledonia	31.50%		285,498
New Zealand	30.80%	27.9	4,822,233
Iraq	30.40%	28	40,222,493
Fiji	30.20%	27.2	896,445
Macau	30.00%		649,335
Hong Kong	29.90%		7,496,981
Bahrain	29.80%	28.2	1,701,575
Canada	29.40%	27.2	37,742,154
Northern Mariana Islands	29.20%		57,559
Australia	29.00%	27.2	25,499,884
Mexico	28.90%	28.1	128,932,753
Malta	28.90%	27.2	441,543
South Africa	28.30%	27.3	59,308,690
Argentina	28.30%	27.7	45,195,774
Chile	28.00%	27.8	19,116,201
Uruguay	27.90%	26.8	3,473,730
Dominica	27.90%	27	71,986
United Kingdom	27.80%	27.3	67,886,011
Syria	27.80%	28.1	17,500,658
Dominican Republic	27.60%	26.7	10,847,910
Algeria	27.40%	26.2	43,851,044
Oman	27.00%	26.9	5,106,626

TABLE 1 Global ranks and trends of obesity—cont'd

Country	Obesity rate	BMI	Population 2020
Tunisia	26.90%	26.8	11,818,619
Palestine	26.80%	27.6	5,101,414
Suriname	26.40%	27.4	586,632
Hungary	26.40%	26.3	9,660,351
Lithuania	26.30%	26.6	2,722,289
Morocco	26.10%	25.6	36,910,560
Israel	26.10%	26.3	8,655,535
Czech Republic	26.00%	26.9	10,708,981
Iran	25.80%	26.2	83,992,949
Costa Rica	25.70%	26.9	5,094,118
Venezuela	25.60%	27.2	28,435,940
Andorra	25.60%	27.5	77,265
Ireland	25.30%	27.5	4,937,786
Vanuatu	25.20%	26.2	307,145
Bulgaria	25.00%	26	6,948,445
Greece	24.90%	27.3	10,423,054
Jamaica	24.70%	27.4	2,961,167
El Salvador	24.60%	27.4	6,486,205
Cuba	24.60%	26.2	11,326,616
Belarus	24.50%	26.6	9,449,323
Croatia	24.40%	25.5	4,105,267
Belize	24.10%	28.9	397,628
Ukraine	24.10%	26	43,733,762
Gibraltar	24.00%	27.5	33,691
Spain	23.80%	26.7	46,754,778
Saint Vincent and the Grenadines	23.70%	27.3	110,940
Nicaragua	23.70%	26.9	6,624,554
Latvia	23.60%	25.8	1,886,198
Montenegro	23.30%	26	628,066

Continued

TABLE 1 Global ranks and trends of obesity—cont'd

Country	Obesity rate	BMI	Population 2020
Russia	23.10%	26.5	145,934,462
Poland	23.10%	26.4	37,846,611
Norway	23.10%	26	5,421,241
Barbados	23.10%	28.7	287,375
Saint Kitts and Nevis	22.90%	29.7	53,199
Guadeloupe	22.90%		400,124
Panama	22.70%	27.1	4,314,767
Haiti	22.70%	24.1	11,402,528
Luxembourg	22.60%	26.5	625,978
Solomon Islands	22.50%	25.5	686,884
Romania	22.50%	25.3	19,237,691
Germany	22.30%	26.3	83,783,942
Colombia	22.30%	25.9	50,882,891
Finland	22.20%	25.9	5,540,720
Brazil	22.10%	25.9	212,559,417
Belgium	22.10%	25.5	11,589,623
Greenland	22.00%		56,770
Taiwan	22.00%	24	23,816,775
Iceland	21.90%	25.9	341,243
Cyprus	21.80%	27	1,207,359
Albania	21.70%	26.1	2,877,797
Georgia	21.70%	27.2	3,989,167
France	21.60%	25.3	65,273,511
Serbia	21.50%	25.8	8,737,371
Honduras	21.40%	26.4	9,904,607
Papua New Guinea	21.30%	25.3	8,947,024
Grenada	21.30%	27	112,523
Guatemala	21.20%	26.5	17,915,568
Estonia	21.20%	25.5	1,326,535

TABLE 1 Global ranks and trends of obesity—cont'd

Country	Obesity rate	BMI	Population 2020
Kazakhstan	21.00%	27.4	18,776,707
Portugal	20.80%	26.2	10,196,709
Sweden	20.60%	25.8	10,099,265
Mongolia	20.60%	26	3,278,290
Slovakia	20.50%	26.5	5,459,642
Netherlands	20.40%	25.4	17,134,872
Paraguay	20.30%	25.8	7,132,538
Slovenia	20.20%	26.9	2,078,938
Bolivia	20.20%	25.9	11,673,021
Armenia	20.20%	26.7	2,963,243
Guyana	20.20%	26.3	786,552
Austria	20.10%	25.4	9,006,398
Isle of Man	20.00%		85,033
Italy	19.90%	26	60,461,826
Azerbaijan	19.90%	27.4	10,139,177
Ecuador	19.90%	27	17,643,054
Saint Lucia	19.70%	29.6	183,627
Peru	19.70%	26.3	32,971,854
Denmark	19.70%	25.3	5,792,202
Switzerland	19.50%	25.3	8,654,622
Botswana	18.90%	24.7	2,351,627
Moldova	18.90%	26.7	4,033,963
Antigua and Barbuda	18.90%	28.1	97,929
Turkmenistan	18.60%	26.4	6,031,200
Trinidad and Tobago	18.60%	28.7	1,399,488
Bosnia and Herzegovina	17.90%	26.1	3,280,819
French Guiana	17.90%		298,682
Namibia	17.20%	24.3	2,540,905
Yemen	17.10%	25.8	29,825,964

Continued

TABLE 1 Global ranks and trends of obesity—cont'd

Country	Obesity rate	BMI	Population 2020
Uzbekistan	16.60%	26.1	33,469,203
Lesotho	16.60%	24.9	2,142,249
Kyrgyzstan	16.60%	26.2	6,524,195
Malaysia	15.60%	25.3	32,365,999
Zimbabwe	15.50%	23.4	14,862,924
Gabon	15.00%	25.5	2,225,734
Tajikistan	14.20%	25.4	9,537,645
Brunei	14.10%	26.2	437,479
Seychelles	14.00%	26.8	98,347
Djibouti	13.50%	23.3	988,000
Mauritania	12.70%	24.8	4,649,658
Sao Tome and Principe	12.40%	24.8	219,159
Cape Verde	11.80%	24.7	555,987
Cameroon	11.40%	24.4	26,545,863
Ghana	10.90%	24.2	31,072,940
Mauritius	10.80%	25.6	1,271,768
Ivory Coast	10.30%	23.6	26,378,274
Gambia	10.30%	24	2,416,668
Thailand	10.00%	24.1	69,799,978
Liberia	9.90%	24	5,057,681
Benin	9.60%	23.4	12,123,200
Republic of the Congo	9.60%	23.3	5,518,087
Nigeria	8.90%	23.4	206,139,589
Senegal	8.80%	23	16,743,927
Sierra Leone	8.70%	22.8	7,976,983
Pakistan	8.60%	23.8	220,892,340
Mali	8.60%	22.8	20,250,833
Maldives	8.60%	25.1	540,544
Tanzania	8.40%	23.1	59,734,218

TABLE 1 Global ranks and trends of obesity—cont'd

Country	Obesity rate	BMI	Population 2020
Togo	8.40%	23.2	8,278,724
Somalia	8.30%	21.9	15,893,222
Angola	8.20%	24.1	32,866,272
Zambia	8.10%	22.6	18,383,955
Equatorial Guinea	8.00%	25.6	1,402,985
Comoros	7.80%	24.1	869,601
Guinea	7.70%	22.7	13,132,795
Central African Republic	7.50%	22.4	4,829,767
Mozambique	7.20%	22.3	31,255,435
Martinique	7.20%		375,265
Kenya	7.10%	23	53,771,296
Indonesia	6.90%	22.9	273,523,615
North Korea	6.80%	21.8	25,778,816
DR Congo	6.70%	22.2	89,561,403
Sudan	6.60%	25.2	43,849,260
South Sudan	6.60%	25.2	11,193,725
Bhutan	6.40%	23.8	771,608
Philippines	6.40%	23.2	109,581,078
China	6.20%	23.9	1,439,323,776
Singapore	6.10%	23.7	5,850,342
Chad	6.10%	22.3	16,425,864
Rwanda	5.80%	22	12,952,218
Malawi	5.80%	22.8	19,129,952
Myanmar	5.80%	22.6	54,409,800
Burkina Faso	5.60%	22.1	20,903,273
Niger	5.50%	21.7	24,206,644
Afghanistan	5.50%	21.6	38,928,346
Burundi	5.40%	20.9	11,890,784
Uganda	5.30%	22	45,741,007

Continued

TABLE 1 Global ranks and trends of obesity—cont'd

Country	Obesity rate	BMI	Population 2020
Madagascar	5.30%	21.1	27,691,018
Laos	5.30%	22.6	7,275,560
Sri Lanka	5.20%	23	21,413,249
Eritrea	5.00%	20.5	3,546,421
South Korea	4.70%	23.9	51,269,185
Ethiopia	4.50%	20.6	114,963,588
Japan	4.30%	22.6	126,476,461
Nepal	4.10%	22.2	29,136,808
India	3.90%	21.9	1,380,004,385
Cambodia	3.90%	21.9	16,718,965
Bangladesh	3.60%	21	164,689,383
Vietnam	2.10%	21.6	97,338,579

http://worldpopulationreview.com/countries/most-obese-countries/.

However, when it comes to the most obese countries in the world according to the Organization for Economic Cooperation and Development (OECD), an organization consisting of 35 of the world's largest economies, the United States ranks number one followed by Mexico and New Zealand with 38.2%, 32.4%, and 30.7% obese people of the adult population, respectively [7]. The highest change in related DALYs and related deaths occurred in Russia between 1990 and 2015 with 26.6% and 42.2%, respectively. The lowest rates were seen in Japan with 1.0% of DALYs and 20.5% of deaths. The greatest burden of DALYs and related deaths was seen in Russia while the lowest rates were observed in the Democratic Republic of Congo, among the 20 most populous countries [1].

Approximately 70% of all elevated BMI-related deaths are secondary to cardiovascular disease and within that group, 60% of all deaths happen in obese people. Generally speaking, obesity is a major risk factor of mortality [11].

Previous studies have argued that there is a higher risk of all-cause mortality with a normal range BMI compared to overweight [7, 12]. However, more recent data suggest that a BMI above 25 increases the risk of death more than a normal BMI. This is from a metaanalysis pool of prospective observational studies. These studies have important significance because they account for cofounding factors and biases from prior studies, such as smoking [13, 14].

Economic concerns

Obesity not only causes health concerns but also put an enormous economic burden on the healthcare systems of the United States and other nations around the world. The biggest contribution to the high costs is the related health consequences obesity brings. As mentioned above, obesity increases the risk of many diseases such as heart disease, cancers, diabetes, kidney disease, and musculoskeletal diseases, and is not only a major risk factor for mortality but also for morbidity and disability. One study estimated the costs of obesity-related health care expenses in 2005 to be $190 billion in the United States, and this had doubled since previous estimates [3, 15]. Thus, treating obesity and its related health care consequences costs billions of dollars in just the United States. Therefore, major global awareness has taken place.

The economic impact of obesity and its related health conditions comes from two majors costs: direct and indirect costs. It is important to know these definitions. The major difference between direct and indirect costs is that only direct costs can be tracked to particular cost objects. It's specific to an objective thing. Indirect costs are the costs that are left over after the direct costs have been computed. The definition of health care-related indirect cost is "resources forgone as a result of a health condition" [16]. In business, examples of direct costs are materials, wages, direct labor, and manufacturing supplies. Examples of indirect costs are production, quality control, and insurances. More specifically related to health and obesity, examples of direct costs are pharmacological therapy, transportation, laboratory, and radiological tests as well as inpatient services, including surgical procedures [17]. Indirect costs are the productivity loss costs due to morbidity and mortality, including wages, the value of the lost work, and insurance [18].

Recent studies demonstrated a relationship between increasing BMI and costs attributable to obesity [19–22]. A systematic review included 23 studies, 11 of which used a top-down population-based approach while the other 12 applied a bottom-up, person-based approach. This review calculated costs attributable to obesity [23]. The population-based approach estimated economic costs by using cumulative data on hospital admissions, morbidity, mortality, general practice consultations, disease-related costs, and other health-related indicators as well as population attributable fraction (PAF) or population attributable risk (PAR) to calculate the costs. The person-based approach analyzed the productivity loss and resources used in individuals with each health problem related to obesity. Seventeen of these studies were from developed countries while six were from developing countries. Based on this, the study identified the economical costs in different countries. For instance, in Brazil, two studies estimated the costs of obesity to be $269.6 million in 2010 [24] versus $1.1 billion per year from 2008 to 2010 [25]. In Germany, the total societal costs of obesity yearly increased from €9.8 million in 2002 to €12.2 million in 2008 [26]. Another study showed the annual cost of obesity in Germany to be €63.0 billion based on claims data from a German health insurance company [27].

A third study to assess the economic burden in Germany in 2008 through a large questionnaire population-based prospective cohort study showed the average 3-month individual health care costs to be €1244 [28]. Moreover, a fourth study calculated the total national health care costs in Germany to be €5.1 billion. This study was done using an OBCOST tool to measure the cost of obesity through its prevalence, incidence, and mortality [29]. In Canada, the annual societal costs were estimated to be CAD $1.0 billion in 2012 according to one study [30].

In Korea, the cost was estimated to be US $1.786 billion in 2005 according to one study, and one study showed that Thailand's estimated cost of obesity in 2009 was $725.3 million [31, 32].

One study from Sweden did a 38-year follow-up of 45,920 Swedish men who were performing mandatory military conscription tests at age 18.7 ± 0.5 years. The study showed that the total lifetime productivity loss due to obesity was €95,400 per man in 2003 [33]. A few studies have reported the per capita costs. Two studies showed that the direct per capita costs of obesity were $2741 in 2005 versus $6899 in 2011, and thus had increased almost three times in 6 years [3, 34].

Another article estimated the direct per capita costs of obesity over a 11.5 year time frame to be $8294.67 in 2006 and $171,482 over a lifetime (>65 years) in 2010 in the United States. When using a Makrov-based microsimulation, the total per capita cost was estimated to be $33,900 and $70,200 over a time frame of 5 and 10 years, respectively, in the United States [35].

Taken together, the cost of obesity is significant and accounts for a large portion of the health care system and societal costs. Because it is estimated that over half the world's population will meet obesity criteria by 2030 [23], these costs will further increase and may in fact have economical burdens globally that far exceed the ones we see today. The economic impact in several countries has already increased over the last few decades. Therefore, this trend is likely to continue unless strategic interventions to prevent obesity are put in place, preferably at a young age. Physical activity and diet control are the two first major steps for prevention of this epidemic and should be emphasized.

Figs. 1–8 are important charts related to the obesity epidemic.

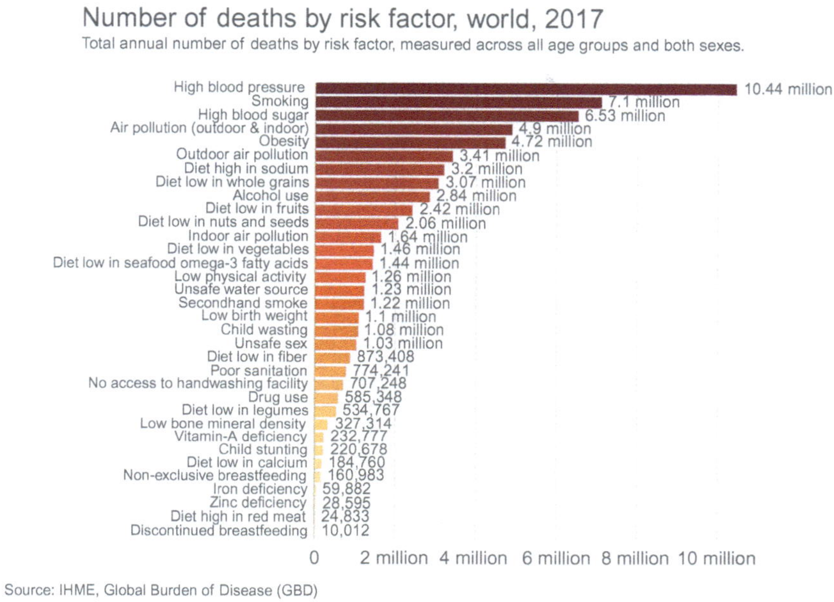

FIG. 1 Number of deaths by risk factors in 2017. Obesity was responsible for 4.7 million premature death each year and was the fifth leading cause.

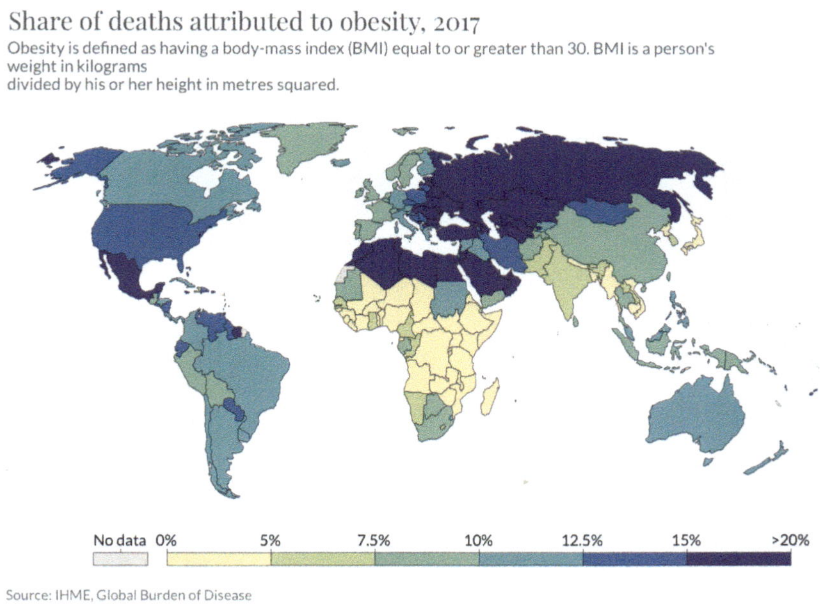

FIG. 2 Share of deaths attributed to obesity in 2017. Worldwide, 8% of deaths were the result of obesity in 2017.

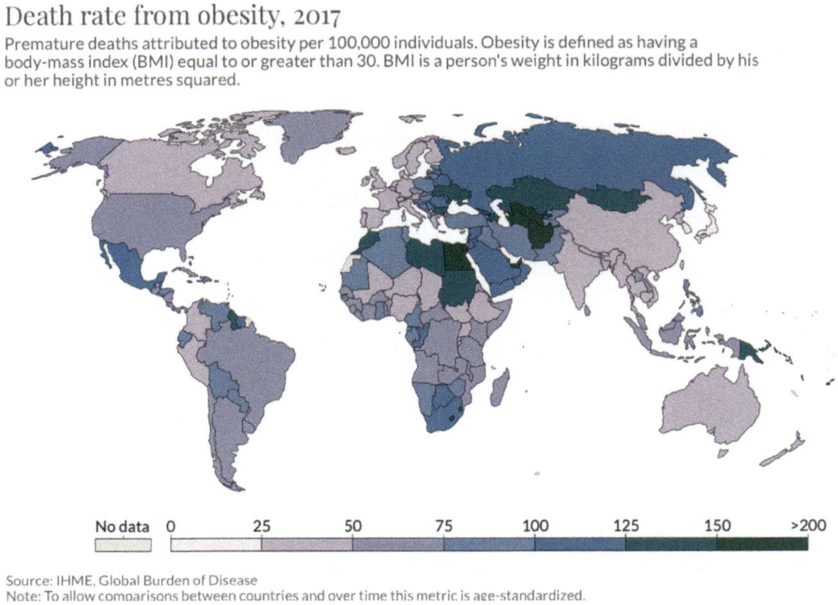

FIG. 3 Death rate from obesity in 2017. There is a 10-fold difference in death rates from obesity across the world.

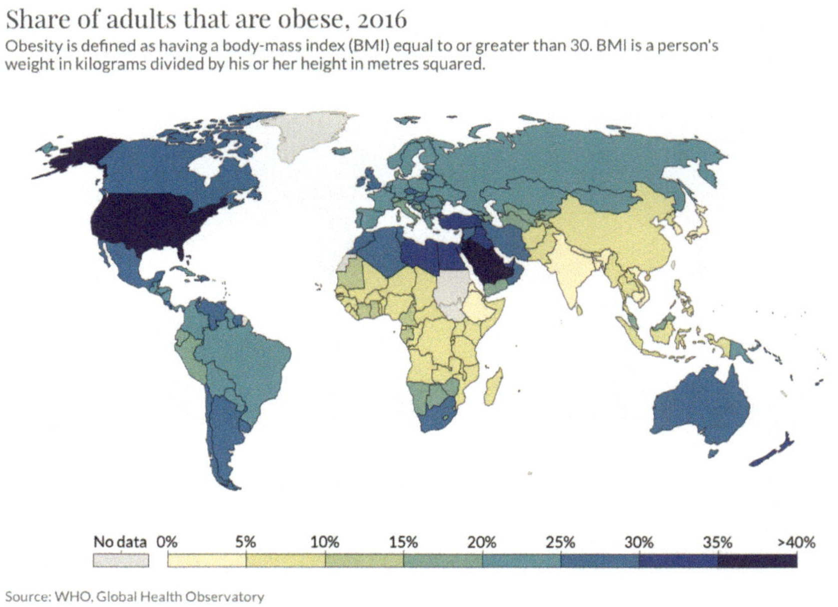

FIG. 4 Shares of adults that were obese in 2016. Worldwide, 13% of adults were obese in 2016.

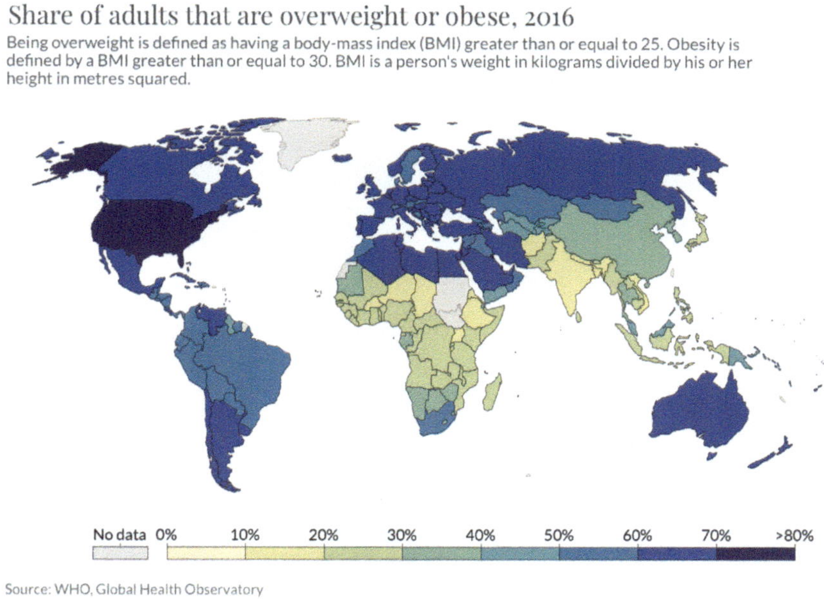

FIG. 5 Share of adults that were overweight or obese in 2016. Worldwide, 39% of adults were overweight or obese.

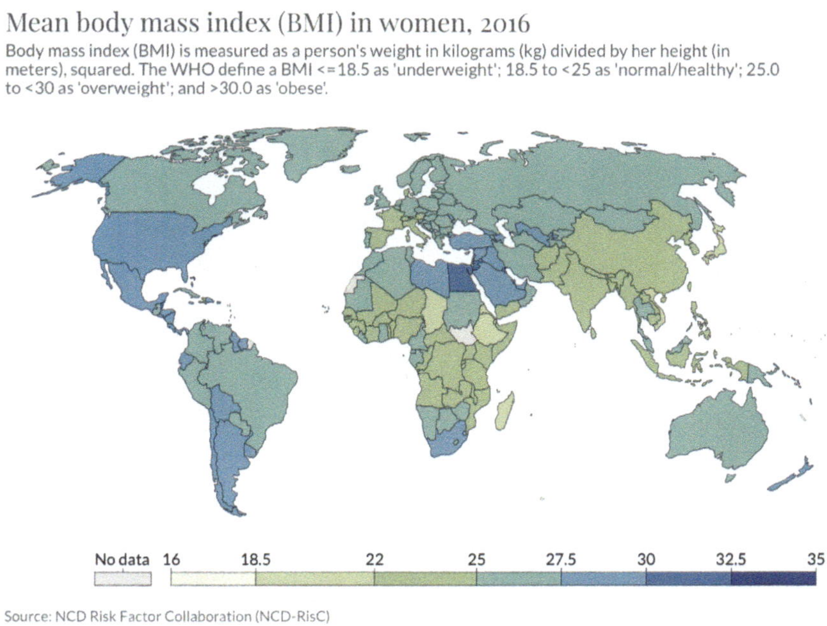

FIG. 6 Mean BMI in women in 2016.

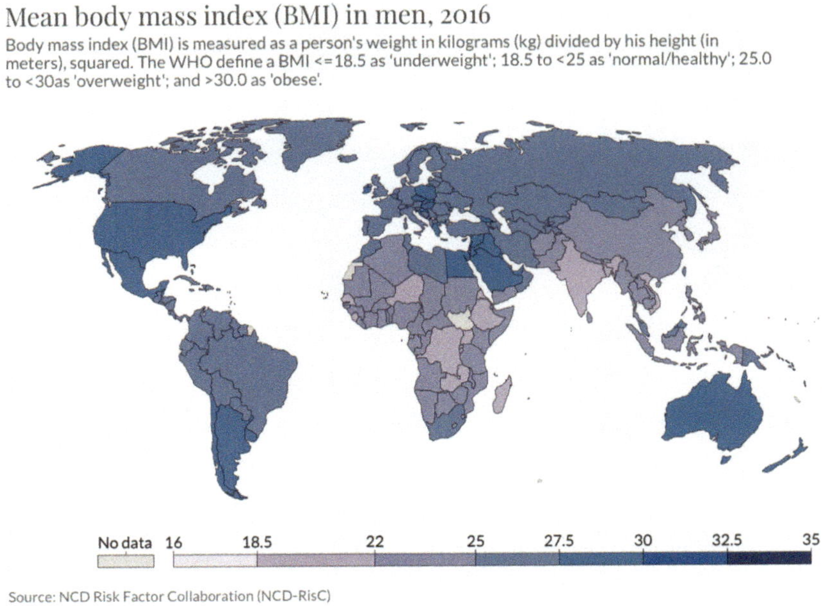

FIG. 7 Mean BMI in men in 2016.

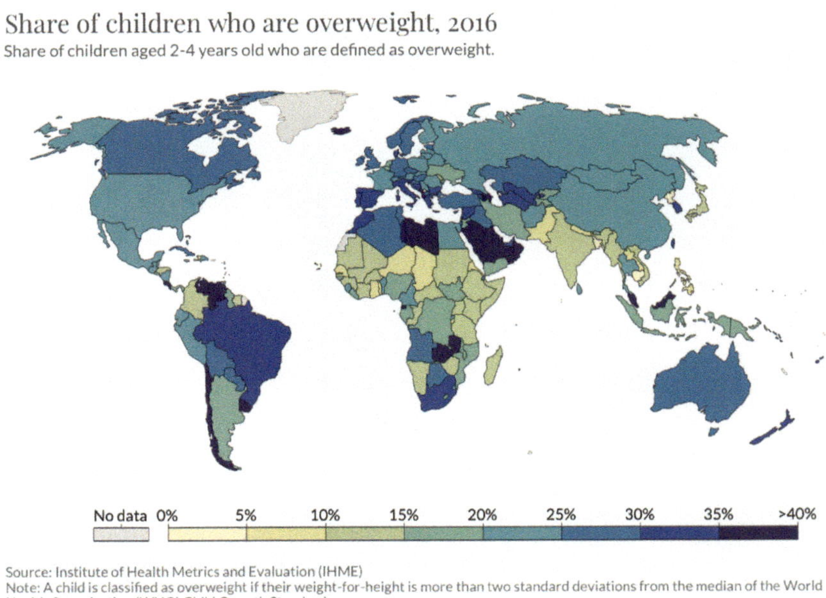

FIG. 8 Share of children who were overweight in 2016.

References

[1] GBD 2015 Obesity Collaborators. Afshin A, Forouzanfar MH, Reitsma MB, Sur P, Estep K, et al. Health effects of overweight and obesity in 195 countries over 25 Years. N Engl J Med 2017 Jul;377(1):13–27. https://doi.org/10.1056/NEJMoa1614362. Epub 2017 Jun 12. PMID: 28604169; PMCID: PMC5477817.

[2] Danaei G, Ding EL, Mozaffarian D, et al. The preventable causes of death in the United States: comparative risk assessment of dietary, lifestyle, and metabolic risk factors. PLoS Med 2009;6:e1000058.

[3] Cawley J, Meyerhoefer C. The medical care costs of obesity: an instrumental variables approach. J Health Econ 2012;31:219–30. https://doi.org/10.1016/j.jhealeco.2011.10.003.

[4] Harvard School of Public Health. Obesity consequences. The high cost of excess weight. Harvard School of Public Health. Available at: https://www.hsph.harvard.edu/obesity-prevention-source/obesity-consequences/.

[5] NCD Risk Factors Collaboration (NCD-RisC). Trends in adult body-mass index in 200 countries from 1975 to 2014: a pooled analysis of 1698 population-based measurement studies with 19·2 million participants. Lancet 2016;387(10026):1377–96.

[6] Ng M, Fleming T, Robinson M, et al. Global, regional, and national prevalence of overweight and obesity in children and adults during 1980–2013: a systematic analysis for the Global Burden of Disease Study 2013. Lancet 2014;384(9945):766–81.

[7] Singh GM, Danaei G, Farzadfar F, et al. The age-specific quantitative effects of metabolic risk factors on cardiovascular diseases and diabetes: a pooled analysis. PLoS One 2013;8(7):e65174.

[8] Lauby-Secretan B, Scoccianti C, Loomis D, Grosse Y, Bianchini F, Straif K. Body fatness and cancer—Viewpoint of the IARC Working Group. N Engl J Med 2016;375(8):794–8.

[9] Gregg EW, Shaw JE. Global Health effects of overweight and obesity. N Engl J Med 2017 Jul;377 (1):80–1. https://doi.org/10.1056/NEJMe1706095. Epub 2017 Jun 12. PMID: 28604226.

[10] World Population Review. Most obese countries 2019. Available at: http://worldpopulationreview.com/countries/most-obese-countries/.

[11] Organization for Economic Co-operation and Development. Available at: http://www.oecd.org/health/health-at-a-glance-19991312.htm.

[12] Flegal KM, Kit BK, Orpana H, Graubard BI. Association of all-cause mortality with overweight and obesity using standard body mass index categories: a systematic review and meta-analysis. JAMA 2013;309(1):71–82.

[13] Global BMI Mortality Collaboration. Body-mass index and all-cause mortality: individual participant-data meta-analysis of 239 prospective studies in four continents. Lancet 2016;388(10046):776–86.

[14] Xia X, Chen W, Li J, et al. Body mass index and risk of breast cancer: a nonlinear dose-response meta-analysis of prospective studies. Sci Rep 2014;4:7480.

[15] Dobbs R, Sawers C, Thompson F, Manyika J, Woetzel JR, Child P, McKenna S, Spatharou A. Overcoming obesity: an initial economic analysis. Jakarta, Indonesia: McKinsey Global Institute; 2014.

[16] USDA. Economic Research Service. Food safety glossary. [Accessed 25 January 2012].

[17] Larg A, Moss JR. Cost-of-illness studies. Pharmacoeconomics 2011;29:653–71. https://doi.org/10.2165/11588380-000000000-00000.

[18] Weinstein M, Siegel J, Gold M, Kamlet M, Russell L. Cost-effectiveness in health and medicine. Oxford, UK: Oxford University Press; 1996.

[19] Andreyeva T, Sturm R, Ringel JS. Moderate and severe obesity have large differences in health care costs. Obes Res 2004;12:1936–43. https://doi.org/10.1038/oby.2004.243.

[20] Dee A, Kearns K, O'Neill C, Sharp L, Staines A, O'Dwyer V, Fitzgerald S, Perry IJ. The direct and indirect costs of both overweight and obesity: a systematic review. BMC Res Notes 2014;7. https://doi.org/10.1186/1756-0500-7-242.

[21] Finkelstein EA, Trogdon JG, Cohen JW, Dietz W. Annual medical spending attributable to obesity: payer-and service-specific estimates. Health Aff 2009;28:w822–31. https://doi.org/10.1377/hlthaff.28.5.w822.

[22] Specchia ML, Veneziano MA, Cadeddu C, Ferriero AM, Mancuso A, Ianuale C, Parente P, Capri S, Ricciardi W. Economic impact of adult obesity on health systems: a systematic review. Eur J Public Health 2015;25:255–62. https://doi.org/10.1093/eurpub/cku170.

[23] Tremmel M, Gerdtham UG, Nilsson PM, Saha S. Economic burden of obesity: a systematic literature review. Int J Environ Res Public Health 2017 Apr;14(4):E435. https://doi.org/10.3390/ijerph14040435 Review. PMID: 28422077; PMCID: PMC5409636.

[24] De Oliveira ML, Santos LM, Da Silva EN. Direct healthcare cost of obesity in Brazil: an application of the cost-of-illness method from the perspective of the public health system in 2011. PLoS One 2015;10:e0121160. https://doi.org/10.1371/journal.pone.0121160.

[25] Bahia L, Coutinho ES, Barufaldi LA, Abreu GA, Malhao TA, De Souza CP, Araujo DV. The costs of overweight and obesity-related diseases in the Brazilian public health system: Cross-sectional study. BMC Public Health 2012;12. https://doi.org/10.1186/1471-2458-12-440.

[26] Lehnert T, Streltchenia P, Konnopka A, Riedel-Heller SG, Konig HH. Health burden and costs of obesity and overweight in Germany: an update. Eur J Health Econ 2015;16:957–67. https://doi.org/10.1007/s10198-014-0645-x.

[27] Effertz T, Engel S, Verheyen F, Linder R. The costs and consequences of obesity in Germany: a new approach from a prevalence and life-cycle perspective. Eur J Health Econ 2016;17:1141–58. https://doi.org/10.1007/s10198-015-0751-4.

[28] Epidemiologische Studie zu Chancen der Verhütung, Früherkennung und optimierten Therapie chronischer Erkrankungen in der älteren Bevölkerung (the ESTHER study).

[29] Lette M, Bemelmans WJ, Breda J, Slobbe LC, Dias J, Boshuizen HC. Health care costs attributable to overweight calculated in a standardized way for three European countries. Eur J Health Econ 2016;17:61–9. https://doi.org/10.1007/s10198-014-0655-8.

[30] Krueger H, Krueger J, Koot J. Variation across Canada in the economic burden attributable to excess weight, tobacco smoking and physical inactivity. Can J Public Health 2015;106: e171–7. https://doi.org/10.17269/cjph.106.4994.

[31] Kang JH, Jeong BG, Cho YG, Song HR, Kim KA. Socioeconomic costs of overweight and obesity in Korean adults. J Korean Med Sci 2011;26:1533–40. https://doi.org/10.3346/jkms.2011.26.12.1533.

[32] Pitayatienanan P, Butchon R, Yothasamut J, Aekplakorn W, Teerawattananon Y, Suksomboon N, Thavorncharoensap M. Economic costs of obesity in Thailand: a retrospective cost-of-illness study. BMC Health Serv Res 2014;14. https://doi.org/10.1186/1472-6963-14-146.

[33] Neovius K, Rehnberg C, Rasmussen F, Neovius M. Lifetime productivity losses associated with obesity status in early adulthood: a population-based study of Swedish men. Appl Health Econ Health Policy 2012;10:309–17. https://doi.org/10.1007/BF03261865.

[34] An R. Health care expenses in relation to obesity and smoking among US adults by gender, race/ethnicity, and age group: 1998–2011. Public Health 2015;129:29–36. https://doi.org/10.1016/j.puhe.2014.11.003.

[35] Su W, Huang J, Chen F, Iacobucci W, Mocarski M, Dall TM, Perreault L. Modeling the clinical and economic implications of obesity using microsimulation. J Med Econ 2015;18:886–97. https://doi.org/10.3111/13696998.2015.1058805.

Chapter 6

The health impact of obesity

Elizabeth Kiwanuka, M.D., Ph.D.
Department of Plastic Surgery, Rhode Island Hospital, Providence, RI, United States

Introduction

Obesity is a significant risk factor for morbidity and mortality from multiple diseases, including diabetes, cardiovascular disease, respiratory disorders, and cancer [1]. Obesity was first acknowledged as a disease by the World Health Organization (WHO) in 1984 and was initially consider a disease of industrialized countries [2]. However, there is a growing body of evidence describing the rising prevalence of obesity throughout the world [2–4]. This represents 18% of overall health expenditures, and much of the cost of obesity comes from related comorbidities [5–10].

Excess body weight is measured by body mass index (BMI; calculated as weight in kg over m^2). Although BMI does not differentiate between bone density, muscle mass, or body fat, it is a general indicator of body fat mass. Adults with a BMI of 23–30kg/m^2 are considered overweight, and a BMI >30 is defined as obesity [11]. Although the relationship between BMI and body fat content varies by age, gender, and ethnicity, the risk of comorbidities has been shown to increase with BMI [12]. Obesity has physical, mental, and social impacts and some of the comorbidities related to overweight include cancers (breast, endometrial, ovarian, colorectal, esophageal, kidney, and prostatic), diabetes and metabolic syndrome, hypertension, cerebrovascular disease, and stroke as well as depression, low self-esteem, mood disorders, discrimination, and social bias [8, 13–21]. There is no specific BMI cutoff for health hazards, and health conditions are often worse in people with a high BMI. This chapter reviews the health impact of obesity and its implications for patients (Table 1).

Physical health impacts

Metabolic syndrome and diabetes

Metabolic syndrome is a constellation of metabolic risk factors, including dyslipidemia, elevated blood pressure, elevated glucose, insulin resistance, and prothrombotic, and proinflammatory states [13, 22]. The metabolic syndrome

Obesity. https://doi.org/10.1016/B978-0-12-818839-2.00006-5

TABLE 1 Impact on health from obesity.

Physical health impacts
• Metabolic syndrome and diabetes • Hypertension and cardiovascular disease • Stroke • Asthma • Sleep apnea • Cancer • Gastroesophageal reflux disease • Musculoskeletal problems • Disability
Impact on mental health
• Low self-esteem and impaired body image • Mood disorders • Eating problems • Sexual health
Impact on social well-being
• Quality of life • Spiritual health impacts

is linked to abdominal obesity, a term used when the waist circumference is more than 102 cm in men or more than 88 cm in women. The prevalence of metabolic syndrome is steadily increasing and leads to a significantly increased risk of cardiovascular disease [23]. People with metabolic syndrome have at least a two-fold increase in risk for cardiovascular disease compared to those without, and the risk for type 2 diabetes is increased five-fold [23–25].

Abdominal obesity and insulin resistance are considered the most critical factors in the development of the metabolic syndrome. Adipose tissue is the largest endocrine organ in the body, and the cytokines released act in autocrine, paracrine, and endocrine manners. In addition, insulin sensitivity fluctuation occurs across the natural life cycle and is noticed during puberty, pregnancy, and during the aging process [26, 27].

The body stores excess nutrients through a process called lipogenesis. In times of calorie deficiency, these nutrients can be used as a supply of energy to organs and tissue through the process of lipolysis. Obesity leads to altered metabolic homeostasis that eventually results in systemic insulin resistance [28]. Insulin sensitivity is affected by body fat distribution, and adipose tissue alters the body's metabolism by secreting hormones, glycerol, and inflammatory mediators [22]. It has been proposed that there is an inadequate response from hypertrophied adipocytes to insulin [29, 30]. However, the mechanism behind the development of insulin resistance is not fully understood.

Diabetes mellitus is a disease characterized by altered carbohydrates, protein, and fat metabolism. The vast majority of people with type 2 diabetes exhibit obesity and insulin resistance [30]. Cell starvation from the lack of intracellular glucose leads to an increase in pancreatic insulin secretion, and prolonged periods of elevated insulin levels lead to dysfunction in its production with ensuing hypoinsulinemia and hyperglycemia [28]. Insulin resistance also leads to elevated fatty acids in the blood and high hepatic glucose production. As discussed above, overweight and obesity are often linked to insulin resistance [31, 32]. Still, diabetes only develops in those individuals who do not have sufficient insulin secretion to match the degree of insulin resistance. In patients with type 2 diabetes, insulin may be high, yet not enough to normalize the level of glycemia [33, 34].

Hypertension and cardiovascular disease

Hypertension is the most common risk factor for stroke, cardiovascular disease, and end-organ damage and is often present in the obese population [35]. Population-based studies consistently demonstrate an increased risk in the development of hypertension among the overweight and obese [36]. Individuals with a BMI of 35–39.9 have a 2.6 times higher risk of developing hypertension as compared to individuals with a healthy BMI. A BMI of 40 and above increases the risk by 4.8 times [37–39].

Obesity-related hypertension is a multifactorial disease with altered hemodynamics, renal dysfunction, and impaired sodium hemostasis. The development of hypertension is believed to be driven by proinflammatory cytokines, resulting in vascular endothelial dysfunction and the progression of arteriosclerotic changes within the vessel wall [40–42].

Obesity has many adverse effects on hemodynamics and cardiovascular function. Obesity leads to increased total blood volume and cardiac workload. With the increase in cardiac filling pressure and volume comes ventricular hypertrophy, and obesity is a risk factor for left ventricular hypertrophy [43]. However, not all obese individuals are hypertensive, suggesting a complicated relationship between obesity and blood pressure that is still not fully understood [44].

Cerebrovascular disease and stroke

Overweight and obesity are associated with progressively increasing risks of ischemic stroke and hemorrhagic stroke [45]. It has been shown that each unit increase in BMI leads to a rise of 4% in the risk of ischemic stroke and 6% for hemorrhagic stroke [12]. In addition, abdominal obesity has been found to be an independent, potent risk factor for ischemic stroke in all race-ethnic groups. The increased risk of stroke may be linked to the higher prevalence of hypertension in obese people. In addition, the prothrombotic and proinflammatory states of obesity may contribute [46].

Respiratory disorders

Obesity is linked to alveolar hypoventilation and obstructive sleep apnea. The obesity-related changes in respiratory function, known as an obesity-hypoventilation syndrome, are most pronounced during sleep [47]. Upper body obesity is a risk factor for obstructive sleep apnea, likely due to obstruction of the larynx. Sleep apnea develops when the muscles controlling tongue movement relax, allowing the base of the tongue to fall back against the posterior pharyngeal wall. This occludes the pharynx and results in a temporary cessation of breathing and transient hypoxia. People suffering from sleep apnea may experience daytime somnolence, pulmonary hypertension, and right-side cardiac failure [48]. Sleep apnea is also associated with an increased risk of myocardial infarction and cerebral infarction [49, 50].

Cancer

It has been established that obesity and overweight are responsible for 14% of all cancer deaths in men and 20% of those in women in the United States [51]. It has been shown that increased BMI is associated with higher risk for many cancers such as endometrial and colorectal cancers, thyroid cancer, ovarian cancer, and postmenopausal breast cancer [52–56]. Although the mechanisms of obesity-related cancer are not known, it has been linked to systemic hormonal and inflammatory changes.

Obesity is a state of caloric excess, and it chronically activates cytokines and growth factor signaling pathways that lead to an increased risk for neoplastic transformation. The altered adipose biology found in people with elevated BMI creates a microenvironment that promotes cancers such as those of the breast and visceral organs. The insulin-cancer hypothesis proposes that prolonged hyperinsulinemia leads to lower levels of insulin growth factor (IGF) binding proteins. This leads to increased levels of bioactive IGF, favoring tumor development [57–59].

The mechanism behind obesity and breast cancer risk is driven by alteration in sex hormones, growth hormones, and cytokines [53]. The adipose tissue expresses sex steroid-metabolizing enzymes that promote the formation of estrogen. After menopause, when ovarian estrogen production is suspended, the fatty tissue becomes the primary source of endogenous estradiol [60–63].

Nonalcoholic fatty liver disease

Nonalcoholic fatty liver disease (NAFLD) is a spectrum of disorders that ultimately leads to cirrhosis and hepatocellular carcinoma [64]. NAFLD is the most common liver disease in the United States, affecting 15–30% of the general population. The ongoing obesity epidemic is believed to play an important role in the increased prevalence of NAFLD [65].

NAFLD is characterized by hepatocellular fat accumulation, and there is a strong association with diabetes mellitus, obesity, and metabolic syndrome. Obesity changes the normal role of the liver in the lipid and energy metabolism, and this leads to a sequence of histopathologic changes. The steatosis is caused by an increase in hepatocellular fat and is proportional to body mass index [66–68].

Given the important role of obesity in the development of NAFLD, addressing the obesity epidemic is critical. The risk of NAFLD is reduced with aggressive strategies for obesity prevention and treatment and should include lifestyle changes as well as medication and surgery [69, 70].

Gastroesophageal reflux disease

Gastroesophageal reflux disease (GERD) often manifests as heartburn, indigestion, coughing coarsens, and bleaching [71]. Studies have shown that an increase in weight is associated with a higher risk for GERD while weight reduction is related to a decrease of reflex symptoms. Obesity is a significant risk factor for GERD, and there are several mechanisms by which obesity causes GERD [72]. Obese patients are more likely to have hiatal hernias compared to nonobese individuals. For each unit increase in BMI, there is a 10% increase in intragastric pressure. The excess visceral fatty tissue may lead to increased intragastric pressure, creating a favorable gradient for reflux to occur. Obesity has also been linked to decreased gastric motility leading to delayed gastric emptying and a higher risk for reflux [73, 74].

Musculoskeletal disease

Although the mechanism is not fully understood, excess fatty tissue is linked to both osteoporosis and osteoarthritis [75]. Osteoporosis is characterized by bone loss and leads to an increased risk for fractures, especially in older adults. In the United States, 30% of postmenopausal women are affected by osteoporosis. Earlier studies showed that increased weight reduces the risk for fractures compared with those with healthy or low BMI. However, recent studies have shown that high BMI is associated with an increased risk for osteoporosis and fractures [76]. The mechanism and link between obesity and osteoporosis are not fully understood. Obesity leads to an increase in bone marrow fat content, and the amount of bone marrow adipocytes is inversely related to bone mineral density. Bone marrow fat and bone tissue interactions are complex and not fully understood.

Obesity leads to an increased risk for the development of osteoarthritis. Obese individuals have a 2.3–4.5 times higher risk as compared to normal-weight individuals to develop osteoarthritis of the knee [77, 78]. The increased risk is due to both mechanical and inflammatory dysfunction [79].

Surgical risks

Obesity complicates surgery and increases perioperative risks [80]. The excess tissue decreases surgical access and can lead to reduced visibility during the operation. Obtaining intraoperative hemostasis may be challenging due to excessive fat in the abdominal wall. There is also a higher risk of difficulty in securing intravenous access.

The obese patient may have impaired healing with subsequent wound dehiscence and infection. Limitations in early postoperative ambulation may lead to an increased risk of deep vein thrombosis and pulmonary emboli [81].

Disability and mortality

Disability is defined as a decreased ability to perform activities of daily living (ADL) due to decreased physical function or mobility, and obesity is shown to limit ADL and work. Not only is obesity linked to disability, but obesity also reduces the likelihood of recovery from disability. Studies have shown that an increase in BMI is associated with an increased risk of subsequent disability.

The net impact of the obesity comorbidities leads to increased mortality. Studies have shown a significant increase in cardiovascular and noncardiovascular mortality associated with obesity as well as cancer. Importantly, studies of patients undergoing gastric bypass surgery for morbid obesity have demonstrated significant reductions in mortality.

Impact on mental health

Studies have indicated that the relationship between weight and mental illness is dose-dependent and that higher BMI increases the risk for psychiatric disorders [82]. However, the relationship between obesity and mental illness is complex and bidirectional. A study of the bariatric surgery population demonstrated that 40–70% of patients have some form of psychiatric illness. A number of cross-sectional studies have found obesity to be linked to mood disorders, including generalized anxiety disorder [83].

The data show the strongest association between obesity and depression, and most of the studies report a significant association [84]. This association is stronger in females and may be due to an inherently higher dissatisfaction with their bodies among females combined with higher social pressures. Some studies have proposed a causal mechanism leading from depression to obesity because increased appetite and weight gain are common symptoms of depression. In addition, medications used to manage mood or anxiety disorders may also lead to weight gain [85–87].

Impact on social well-being

The stigma of obesity has been documented to affect many aspects of life, and obesity has been shown to be associated with negative social consequences [88].

Obese individuals have reported job discrimination, insulting comments, and derogatory media representations. In a study by Carr and Friedman, 40–50% of persons classified as obese experienced significant discrimination due to their weight.

Quality of life

Quality of life encompasses both positive and negative metrics and helps capture the impact of the disease on physical, mental, and social well-being. This widespread defection is especially useful to gauge wellness in people with obesity. In addition, sexual dysfunction is not uncommon among obese individuals. In men, obesity is associated with lower sexual satisfaction and an increase in sexual dysfunction [89].

Obesity is often comorbid with chronic pain caused by osteoarthritis, fibromyalgia, lower back pain, and the presence of pain that can affect the quality of life [90, 91].

Spiritual health impacts

Spiritual well-being is believed to decrease emotional eating. There is limited evidence that indicates that emotional eating contributes to a higher caloric intact and weight gain. Religion and spirituality have also been shown to have a role in the treatment of eating disorders [91].

References

[1] Casazza K, et al. Myths, presumptions, and facts about obesity. N Engl J Med 2013;368(5): 446–54.

[2] James PT. Obesity: the worldwide epidemic. Clin Dermatol 2004;22(4):276–80.

[3] Ogden CL, et al. The epidemiology of obesity. Gastroenterology 2007;132(6):2087–102.

[4] Brownell KD, et al. The public health and economic benefits of taxing sugar-sweetened beverages. N Engl J Med 2009;361(16):1599–605.

[5] Yun S, et al. A comparison of national estimates of obesity prevalence from the behavioral risk factor surveillance system and the National Health and Nutrition Examination Survey. Int J Obes (Lond) 2006;30(1):164–70.

[6] Wang Y, et al. Will all Americans become overweight or obese? Estimating the progression and cost of the US obesity epidemic. Obesity (Silver Spring) 2008;16(10):2323–30.

[7] Dee A, et al. The direct and indirect costs of both overweight and obesity: a systematic review. BMC Res Notes 2014;7:242.

[8] Li Q, et al. Prevalence and healthcare costs of obesity-related comorbidities: evidence from an electronic medical records system in the United States. J Med Econ 2015;18(12):1020–8.

[9] Specchia ML, et al. Economic impact of adult obesity on health systems: a systematic review. Eur J Public Health 2015;25(2):255–62.

[10] Tremmel M, et al. Economic burden of obesity: a systematic literature review. Int J Environ Res Public Health 2017;14(4).

[11] Goh VHH, et al. Are BMI and other anthropometric measures appropriate as indices for obesity? A study in an Asian population. J Lipid Res 2004;45(10):1892–8.
[12] Kurth T, et al. Body mass index and the risk of stroke in men. Arch Intern Med 2002; 162(22):2557–62.
[13] Abete I, et al. Obesity and the metabolic syndrome: role of different dietary macronutrient distribution patterns and specific nutritional components on weight loss and maintenance. Nutr Rev 2010;68(4):214–31.
[14] Anand G, Katz PO. Gastroesophageal reflux disease and obesity. Gastroenterol Clin North Am 2010;39(1):39–46.
[15] Khan A, et al. Impact of obesity treatment on gastroesophageal reflux disease. World J Gastroenterol 2016;22(4):1627–38.
[16] Nadaleto BF, Herbella FA, Patti MG. Gastroesophageal reflux disease in the obese: pathophysiology and treatment. Surgery 2016;159(2):475–86.
[17] Corley DA, et al. Abdominal obesity and body mass index as risk factors for Barrett's esophagus. Gastroenterology 2007;133(1):34–41.
[18] Hurt RT, et al. Obesity and inflammation: should the principles of immunonutrition be applied to this disease process? Curr Gastroenterol Rep 2007;9(4):305–8.
[19] Matheson PJ, et al. Obesity-induced hepatic hypoperfusion primes for hepatic dysfunction after resuscitated hemorrhagic shock. Surgery 2009;146(4):739–48.
[20] de Koning L, et al. Waist circumference and waist-to-hip ratio as predictors of cardiovascular events: meta-regression analysis of prospective studies. Eur Heart J 2007;28(7):850–6.
[21] Spradley FT. Metabolic abnormalities and obesity's impact on the risk for developing preeclampsia. Am J Physiol Regul Integr Comp Physiol 2017;312(1):R5–R12.
[22] Gluvic Z, et al. Link between metabolic syndrome and insulin resistance. Curr Vasc Pharmacol 2017;15(1):30–9.
[23] Engin A. The definition and prevalence of obesity and metabolic syndrome. Adv Exp Med Biol 2017;960:1–17.
[24] Despres JP, et al. Abdominal obesity and the metabolic syndrome: contribution to global cardiometabolic risk. Arterioscler Thromb Vasc Biol 2008;28(6):1039–49.
[25] Trepanowski JF, et al. Effect of alternate-day fasting on weight loss, weight maintenance, and cardioprotection among metabolically healthy obese adults. JAMA Intern Med 2017; 177(7):930.
[26] Kershaw EE, Flier JS. Adipose tissue as an endocrine organ. J Clin Endocrinol Metab 2004; 89(6):2548–56.
[27] Goossens GH. The metabolic phenotype in obesity: fat mass, body fat distribution, and adipose tissue function. Obes Facts 2017;10(3):207–15.
[28] Yazici D, Sezer H. Insulin resistance, obesity and lipotoxicity. Adv Exp Med Biol 2017;960:277–304.
[29] Samson SL, Garber AJ. Metabolic syndrome. Endocrinol Metab Clin North Am 2014; 43(1):1–23.
[30] Guo S. Insulin signaling, resistance, and the metabolic syndrome: insights from mouse models into disease mechanisms. J Endocrinol 2014;220(2):T1–t23.
[31] Kahn SE. The relative contributions of insulin resistance and beta-cell dysfunction to the pathophysiology of type 2 diabetes. Diabetologia 2003;46(1):3–19.
[32] DeFronzo RA. Pathogenesis of type 2 diabetes mellitus. Med Clin North Am 2004;88(4): 787–835 [ix].
[33] Nolan CJ, et al. Insulin resistance as a physiological defense against metabolic stress: implications for the management of subsets of type 2 diabetes. Diabetes 2015;64(3): 673–86.

[34] Wong J, Tabet E. The introduction of insulin in type 2 diabetes mellitus. Aust Fam Physician 2015;44(5):278–83.
[35] Dhaliwal SS, Welborn TA. Central obesity and multivariable cardiovascular risk as assessed by the Framingham prediction scores. Am J Cardiol 2009;103(10):1403–7.
[36] Lee CMY, et al. Indices of abdominal obesity are better discriminators of cardiovascular risk factors than BMI: a meta-analysis. J Clin Epidemiol 2008;61(7):646–53.
[37] Larsson B, et al. Abdominal adipose tissue distribution, obesity, and risk of cardiovascular disease and death: 13 year follow up of participants in the study of men born in 1913. BMJ 1984;288(6428):1401–4.
[38] Gregg EW. Secular trends in cardiovascular disease risk factors according to body mass index in US adults. JAMA 2005;293(15):1868.
[39] Burke V. Obesity in childhood and cardiovascular risk. Clin Exp Pharmacol Physiol 2006; 33(9):831–7.
[40] Seravalle G, Grassi G. Obesity and hypertension. Pharmacol Res 2017;122:1–7.
[41] Virdis A, et al. Microvascular endothelial dysfunction in obesity and hypertension. Curr Pharm Des 2013;19(13):2382–9.
[42] Engin A. Endothelial dysfunction in obesity. Adv Exp Med Biol 2017;960:345–79.
[43] Landsberg L, et al. Obesity-related hypertension: pathogenesis, cardiovascular risk, and treatment: a position paper of the Obesity Society and the American Society of Hypertension. J Clin Hypertens (Greenwich) 2013;15(1):14–33.
[44] Susic D, Varagic J. Obesity: a perspective from hypertension. Med Clin North Am 2017; 101(1):139–57.
[45] Mitchell AB, et al. Obesity increases risk of ischemic stroke in young adults. Stroke 2015; 46(6):1690–2.
[46] Aparicio HJ, et al. Overweight, obesity, and survival after stroke in the Framingham heart study. J Am Heart Assoc 2017;6(6).
[47] Robinson PD. Obesity and its impact on the respiratory system. Paediatr Respir Rev 2014; 15(3):219–26.
[48] Wouters EFM. Obesity and metabolic abnormalities in chronic obstructive pulmonary disease. Ann Am Thorac Soc 2017;14(Suppl. 5):S389–94.
[49] Semelka M, Wilson J, Floyd R. Diagnosis and treatment of obstructive sleep apnea in adults. Am Fam Physician 2016;94(5):355–60.
[50] Tuomilehto H, Seppa J, Uusitupa M. Obesity and obstructive sleep apnea—clinical significance of weight loss. Sleep Med Rev 2013;17(5):321–9.
[51] De Pergola G, Silvestris F. Obesity as a major risk factor for cancer. J Obes 2013;2013:291546.
[52] Cao Y, Giovannucci E. Obesity and prostate cancer. Recent Results Cancer Res 2016;208:137–53.
[53] Fortner RT, et al. Obesity and breast cancer. Recent Results Cancer Res 2016;208:43–65.
[54] James FR, et al. Obesity in breast cancer—what is the risk factor? Eur J Cancer 2015; 51(6):705–20.
[55] Kyrgiou M, et al. Adiposity and cancer at major anatomical sites: umbrella review of the literature. BMJ 2017;356:j477.
[56] Shaw E, et al. Obesity and endometrial cancer. Recent Results Cancer Res 2016;208:107–36.
[57] Cozzo AJ, Fuller AM, Makowski L. Contribution of adipose tissue to development of cancer. Compr Physiol 2017;8(1):237–82.
[58] Iyengar NM, et al. Obesity and cancer mechanisms: tumor microenvironment and inflammation. J Clin Oncol 2016;34(35):4270–6.
[59] Nimptsch K, Pischon T. Obesity biomarkers, metabolism and risk of cancer: an epidemiological perspective. Recent Results Cancer Res 2016;208:199–217.

[60] Engin A. Obesity-associated breast cancer: analysis of risk factors. Adv Exp Med Biol 2017;960:571–606.

[61] Jiralerspong S, Goodwin PJ. Obesity and breast cancer prognosis: evidence, challenges, and opportunities. J Clin Oncol 2016;34(35):4203–16.

[62] Picon-Ruiz M, et al. Obesity and adverse breast cancer risk and outcome: mechanistic insights and strategies for intervention. CA Cancer J Clin 2017;67(5):378–97.

[63] Zahid H, Simpson ER, Brown KA. Inflammation, dysregulated metabolism and aromatase in obesity and breast cancer. Curr Opin Pharmacol 2016;31:90–6.

[64] Ahmed A, Wong RJ, Harrison SA. Nonalcoholic fatty liver disease review: diagnosis, treatment, and outcomes. Clin Gastroenterol Hepatol 2015;13(12):2062–70.

[65] Chalasani N, et al. The diagnosis and management of nonalcoholic fatty liver disease: practice guidance from the American Association for the Study of Liver Diseases. Hepatology 2018; 67(1):328–57.

[66] Jung UJ, Choi MS. Obesity and its metabolic complications: the role of adipokines and the relationship between obesity, inflammation, insulin resistance, dyslipidemia and nonalcoholic fatty liver disease. Int J Mol Sci 2014;15(4):6184–223.

[67] Milic S, Lulic D, Stimac D. Non-alcoholic fatty liver disease and obesity: biochemical, metabolic and clinical presentations. World J Gastroenterol 2014;20(28):9330–7.

[68] Polyzos SA, Kountouras J, Mantzoros CS. Obesity and nonalcoholic fatty liver disease: from pathophysiology to therapeutics. Metabolism 2019;92:82–97.

[69] Rinella ME. Nonalcoholic fatty liver disease: a systematic review. JAMA 2015;313(22): 2263–73.

[70] Woo Baidal JA, Lavine JE. The intersection of nonalcoholic fatty liver disease and obesity. Sci Transl Med 2016;8(323):323rv1.

[71] Gorodner V, et al. Gastroesophageal reflux disease and morbid obesity: evaluation and treatment. Updates Surg 2018;70(3):331–7.

[72] Richter JE, Rubenstein JH. Presentation and epidemiology of gastroesophageal reflux disease. Gastroenterology 2018;154(2):267–76.

[73] Sethi S, Richter JE. Diet and gastroesophageal reflux disease: role in pathogenesis and management. Curr Opin Gastroenterol 2017;33(2):107–11.

[74] Tack J, Pandolfino JE. Pathophysiology of gastroesophageal reflux disease. Gastroenterology 2018;154(2):277–88.

[75] Collins KH, et al. Obesity, metabolic syndrome, and musculoskeletal disease: common inflammatory pathways suggest a central role for loss of muscle integrity. Front Physiol 2018;9:112.

[76] Godziuk K, et al. The impact of sarcopenic obesity on knee and hip osteoarthritis: a scoping review. BMC Musculoskelet Disord 2018;19(1):271.

[77] Sartori-Cintra AR, Aikawa P, Cintra DE. Obesity versus osteoarthritis: beyond the mechanical overload. Einstein (Sao Paulo) 2014;12(3):374–9.

[78] Bookman JS, et al. Obesity: the modifiable risk factor in total joint arthroplasty. Orthop Clin North Am 2018;49(3):291–6.

[79] Oliveira MC, Vullings J, van de Loo FAJ. Osteoporosis and osteoarthritis are two sides of the same coin paid for obesity. Nutrition 2019;70:110486.

[80] Tewari N, et al. Obesity-related insulin resistance: implications for the surgical patient. Int J Obes (Lond) 2015;39(11):1575–88.

[81] Daniel Guerron A, Portenier DD. Patient selection and surgical management of high-risk patients with morbid obesity. Surg Clin North Am 2016;96(4):743–62.

[82] Avila C, et al. An overview of links between obesity and mental health. Curr Obes Rep 2015; 4(3):303–10.

[83] McElroy SL. Obesity in patients with severe mental illness: overview and management. J Clin Psychiatry 2009;70(Suppl. 3):12–21.
[84] Taylor VH, et al. An overview of treatments for obesity in a population with mental illness. Can J Psychiatry 2012;57(1):13–20.
[85] Mizock L. The double stigma of obesity and serious mental illnesses: promoting health and recovery. Psychiatr Rehabil J 2012;35(6):466–9.
[86] Taylor VH, et al. Beyond pharmacotherapy: understanding the links between obesity and chronic mental illness. Can J Psychiatry 2012;57(1):5–12.
[87] Berkowitz RI, Fabricatore AN. Obesity, psychiatric status, and psychiatric medications. Psychiatr Clin North Am 2011;34(4):747–64.
[88] Doll HA, Petersen SE, Stewart-Brown SL. Obesity and physical and emotional well-being: associations between body mass index, chronic illness, and the physical and mental components of the SF-36 questionnaire. Obes Res 2000;8(2):160–70.
[89] Taylor VH, et al. The impact of obesity on quality of life. Best Pract Res Clin Endocrinol Metab 2013;27(2):139–46.
[90] Hebebrand J, Herpertz-Dahlmann B. Psychological and psychiatric aspects of pediatric obesity. Child Adolesc Psychiatr Clin N Am 2009;18(1):49–65.
[91] Mannucci E, et al. Clinical and psychological correlates of health-related quality of life in obese patients. Health Qual Life Outcomes 2010;8:90.

Chapter 7

Psychosocial factors and outcomes of obesity

Jacqueline Chu, B.A.[a] and Raman Mehrzad, M.D., M.H.L., M.B.A.[b]
[a]*The Ohio State University College of Medicine, Columbus, OH, United States,* [b]*Department of Plastic and Reconstructive Surgery, Rhode Island Hospital, The Warren Alpert Medical School of Brown University, Providence, RI, United States*

Introduction

Multiple large cross-sectional epidemiological studies have demonstrated the presence of an association between obesity and mental health disorders, including depression, anxiety, eating disorders, and substance abuse. This association has been seen for both adults and children in the United States and around the world [1–3]. However, much work is still being done to further understand and elucidate this relationship. This chapter aims to describe the psychosocial contributions and consequences of obesity.

Association between obesity and psychosocial functioning

The association between obesity and psychosocial functioning has been shown to be bidirectional, such that certain psychosocial factors can contribute to obesity and obesity can impact psychosocial functioning. This effect has been noted in multiple studies, including prospective cohort and metaanalyses [4–8]. For example, Luppino et al. (2010) conducted a meta-analysis of longitudinal studies on depression and obesity, reporting that obesity increased the risk of depression with an odds ratio of 1.55, and depression increased the risk of obesity with a similar odds ratio of 1.58 [8]. The following sections will describe the connection between obesity and a number of psychosocial conditions. What will be clear through analysis of the current scope of obesity research is the vicious cycle that persists between psychosocial functioning and obesity.

Bidirectional association between depression and obesity

As acknowledged previously, depression and obesity seem to have a bidirectional relationship in both the adult and adolescent populations [4–10]. For both

Obesity. https://doi.org/10.1016/B978-0-12-818839-2.00007-7

populations, the female gender seems to increase the strength of association in either direction between obesity and depression. However, it appears that the strength of association is equivalent for obesity leading to depression and depression leading to obesity for adults; the strength of association is much more significant for depression leading to obesity in adolescents [7, 8, 10].

Much of the current research is dedicated to understanding this relationship through the identification of mediators and moderators. One well-studied area of research is the metabolic changes and dysfunction associated with both obesity and depression. Hamer et al. (2012) conducted a longitudinal study of 3851 adults from the English Longitudinal Study of Aging cohort, and found that individuals who were obese but metabolically healthy, as determined through the analysis of metabolic biomarkers such as blood pressure and cholesterol, did not have increased risk of depression [11]. This is perhaps consistent with findings seen in other longitudinal studies that have noted that being overweight, but not obese, was often not associated or weakly associated with increased depression risk [8, 10]. An in-depth discussion of the metabolic changes that link depression and obesity is beyond the scope of this work, but is reviewed by Hryhorczuk et al. (2013) [12]. In brief, obesity, particularly central adiposity, predisposes to the production of a milieu of stress and proinflammatory hormones that not only promote metabolic dysregulation in the form of insulin and leptin resistance, but also alter brain chemistry, leading to depressed or anxious moods. Conversely, depression and anxiety predispose individuals to the consumption of high-fat and high-sugar foods to combat negative feelings, likely through the activation of reward pathways. This leads to a vicious cycle, as these types of foods then lead to adiposity and metabolic dysfunction.

Genetic factors may also account for part of the relationship between depression and obesity. A systematic review of genome-wide association studies identified 24 genes that are shared by cardiometabolic diseases and major depressive disorders. Of note, many of the genes identified were linked to the hypothalamic–pituitary–adrenal axis, which is related to cortisol production and stress responses; this is in line with studies on the metabolic mediators of depression and obesity described above [13]. In addition, genetic factors may partially explain the stronger association between obesity and depression in women. Several studies have demonstrated differential effects of certain gene polymorphisms between men and women [14–17]. Tyrrell et al. (2019), for example, used Mendelian randomization of the United Kingdom (UK) Biobank to test the association of a 73-gene variant BMI risk score and the development of depression. For individuals with a risk score of 1 standard deviation above average, the odds ratio of depression for men was 1.08 while the odds ratio of depression for women was 1.21 [17]. This indicates that there is potentially a genetic component that influences the effect of the environment on mood and weight for women that is not quite as impactful for men.

Behavior has also been shown to have a strong influence on the relationship between depression and obesity and can also partially explain gender differences. Women, regardless of weight, have been shown to have greater body-weight dissatisfaction than men, and obese women are more likely than normal-weight women to be dissatisfied with their weight [18, 19]. Body-weight dissatisfaction is, in turn, associated with disordered eating and depression [20, 21]. In addition, multiple studies have noted the effect of physical and social activities on the development of obesity or depression [22–25]. Carroll et al. (2010) found that women, not men, who decreased from the "high vigorous activity" category had increased odds of depression at follow-up [23]. A longitudinal study by Vittengl (2018) confirmed these results in middle-aged women and showed that the effects of physical and social activity were bidirectional and mediated the development of obesity from depression and depression from obesity [24].

Psychosocial functioning as a risk factor for obesity

Stressors, especially those early in life, can have a tremendous impact on our health and well-being, both immediately and in the future. The following section summarizes the evidence connecting stressful life events to obesity development.

Childhood interpersonal violence

Extensive research has established a connection between interpersonal violence during childhood and the development of obesity in adulthood. A meta-analysis conducted by Danese and Tan (2014) on 41 studies demonstrated an odds ratio of 1.36 in terms of the likelihood of developing obesity if interpersonal violence was present during childhood [26]. Furthermore, longitudinal research has shown that the direction of causality is such that interpersonal violence precedes obesity development. For example, a prospective study by Bentley and Widom followed children with court-confirmed cases of abuse and nonabused matched controls for 30 years. The authors noted that children with physical abuse had significantly higher BMI in adulthood than controls; this trend was not seen in children with sexual abuse [27]. Similar results are reflected in Shin and Miller (2012), a longitudinal cohort study of the AddHealth cohort. They found that children who experienced childhood neglect and abuse had a faster average BMI growth trajectory compared to children who experienced no maltreatment [28].

The relationship between interpersonal violence by peers during childhood, such as bullying, and obesity development has been especially well studied. In a meta-analysis of 30 studies including 55,231 overweight and 58,520 obese youths by van Geel et al. (2014), the overall odds ratios were 1.19 and 1.51 for overweight and obese individuals, respectively, in terms of their risk of being victims of bullying [29]. No difference in ORs was noted between boys and girls. Kukaswadia et al. (2011) also noted that obese males were more likely to be victims of physical bullying while obese males were more likely targets of relational bullying [30]. Interestingly, both obese boys and obese girls have also been shown to have increased odds of being bullies themselves, with this effect seen more strongly in obese males [30–32]. While it may appear that weight stigmatization and discrimination are the causes of bullying and other forms of interpersonal violence, multiple large longitudinal studies have demonstrated that childhood bullying in fact predisposes to obesity in adolescence and adulthood. Of note, this effect was still seen even when stratifying or controlling for baseline BMI and strengthened with increased chronicity of bullying. In addition, this effect tended to be stronger in females in comparison to males [33–35]. In order to explain this effect, Sutin et al. (2016) noted that depressive symptoms served as a mediator for the relationship between bullying and obesity development, potentially indicating that the stress from victimization leads to maladaptive coping and emotional processing [36]. Indeed, weight-related teasing has been associated with greater body dissatisfaction and emotional eating/binge eating among adolescent girls [37, 38].

PTSD

The connections between PTSD and obesity further demonstrate the impact of life stressors on obesity development. In a cross-sectional study by Brewerton et al. (2015), a random sample of 3012 women, part of the National Women's Study, was surveyed for the occurrence of crime victimization experiences, PTSD, depression, and bulimia nervosa. A lifetime diagnosis of extreme obesity (BMI greater than or equal to 40) was strongly associated with a diagnosis of PTSD, either at the time of the survey or in the past and with bingeing, purging, and bulimia [39]. Similar results were seen in studies on veterans with PTSD, with increased rates of obesity and emotional eating [40, 41]. A longitudinal study by Kubzansky et al. (2014) was able to establish a temporal link between PTSD and obesity. This study was able to demonstrate that, among women diagnosed with PTSD and who had at least four symptoms of PTSD, BMI rose faster after PTSD onset than prior to PTSD onset, indicating that PTSD likely led to weight gain and subsequent obesity. This effect was maintained even after adjusting for covariates such as depression [42]. Potential theories explaining the association between PTSD and obesity are related to the role of sympathetic nervous system activation and the release of stress hormones in altering brain function, leading to changes in appetite and eating behaviors [43]. This is certainly consistent with the studies mentioned above linking PTSD with eating disorders and emotional eating.

Childhood high-risk behaviors/substance abuse

Studies on adolescents have shown that obesity and substance use are positively correlated. Multiple studies have noted an association between increasing BMI during adolescence and cigarette smoking, but not alcohol or other substances

[44–51]. A collection of prospective studies using the National Longitudinal Study of Adolescent Health cohort, conducted by Huang et al., used latent class analysis to divide this population into groups with shared trajectories or behaviors related to obesity, high-risk behaviors, and substance use in order to identify relationships tying these high-risk behaviors to the development of obesity. In all these studies, groups with a greater prevalence of substance use and other behaviors associated with poor psychosocial functioning were associated with higher rates of obesity or high BMI trajectories [47–50]. The authors of these studies argue that adolescents who initiate these high-risk behaviors are also more likely to initiate unhealthy behaviors that lead to obesity [47]. Pasch et al. (2011) confirmed these conclusions through a bidirectional analysis of participants from two prospective cohorts, which also demonstrated that the presence of substance use was indicative of obesity in the future while no association was found for the reverse hypothesis [51]. This is consistent with the previous findings described on childhood interpersonal violence, in which stressors early in life lead to maladaptive psychological and biological processes that predispose to high-risk behaviors and obesity.

However, these studies do not discount the possibility of obesity contributing to worsening psychosocial functioning through weight stigmatization, leading to negative coping strategies such as substance use. Lanza et al. (2015) found that out of four psychosocial classes, there was a larger proportion of obese individuals in the maladjusted class, the group with the second-highest rate of cigarette and marijuana smoking [49]. Indeed, there may be a bidirectionality to the relationship between substance use and obesity in adolescents–childhood stressors lead to maladaptive behaviors that cause weight gain and obesity, which in turn lead to stigmatization and internalization of weight stigma that predisposes to substance use and other high-risk adolescent behaviors. In support of this trend, a prospective study of 1047 children aged 7–11 conducted by Zuba and Warschburger showed that weight teasing and resulting weight bias internalization were associated with emotional and conduct problems 2 years later [52].

ADHD

Two metaanalyses by Cortese and Nigg, both in 2016, demonstrated a link between childhood ADHD and obesity, with the strength of the association greater for adults than for adolescents [53, 54]. In addition, several longitudinal studies have concluded that ADHD symptoms likely preceded obesity [55–57]. For example, in a cohort of 207 men diagnosed with childhood ADHD, Cortese et al. (2013) demonstrated an odds ratio of 2.99 in terms of the likelihood that individuals with childhood ADHD will be obese in adulthood [56]. Similarly, Khalife et al. (2014) followed a cohort of 8106 children from age 7–8 to age 16 who were part of the Northern Finland Birth Cohort 1986, and demonstrated a smaller odds ratio of 1.91. This effect was seen even after controlling for baseline BMI, and no similar association was seen in the reverse causal direction [55].

There are multiple theories that attempt to explain the association between ADHD and obesity, including genetic differences, altered eating habits, sleep patterns, inflammation, reward pathways, etc., and it is likely that all these factors play at least a small role [58]. Overall, the mechanisms underlying this association are still unclear and are worthy of further study.

Obesity as a risk factor for worsened psychosocial functioning

Studies reported the poorer overall quality of life in obese individuals, with contributions from health, psychological, and social factors. Obese individuals face greater social stigma and internalization of negative social biases, have poorer health-related QoL even after excluding major chronic conditions linked to obesity, and are at increased risk of mental illness [59]. This section will cover the major psychosocial consequences of obesity that contribute to a decreased quality of life in obese individuals.

Weight-based discrimination

Evidence of weight-based discrimination is present in almost every social domain, leading to differential opportunities in domains such as employment, health care, and relationships [60]. Obese individuals were less likely to be chosen for employment or promotion and more likely to have their accomplishments underestimated [61, 62]. Health care professionals have been shown to have negative explicit and implicit biases regarding the obese, with beliefs that obese individuals are less adherent, lazier, and less disciplined. Associated with these stereotypes, health care professionals spend less time with obese individuals, use less patient-centered communication, and were more likely to recommend weight loss for obese patients' health complaints rather than do additional diagnostic work-up [63, 64]. Obesity affects social relationships as well, with studies demonstrating greater feelings of disgust toward obese individuals and decreased perceived attractiveness [65, 66]. In addition, overweight and obese women were reported to have decreased relationship satisfaction and believe that their partners will end their relationships [67].

Eating disorders

Body image dissatisfaction is a well-studied risk factor for eating disorders, including anorexia, bulimia, and binge eating [18, 68], and individuals who are obese, especially women, have been shown to exhibit higher body dissatisfaction in comparison to normal-weight individuals [19]. In addition, the prevalence of individuals with comorbid obesity and eating disorders has been shown to be increasing, lending support to the theory that obesity and eating disorders are linked [69, 70].

Multiple studies have demonstrated that obesity, particularly the stigma of obesity, is associated with the development of unhealthy weight-control habits and eating disorders [71–74]. Common risk factors between eating disorders—particularly bulimia and binge eating—and obesity have been identified; both eating disorders and obesity are linked to body image dissatisfaction, concerns with weight, weight teasing by peers or family, and dieting or weight-control behaviors [75, 76]. However, studies have demonstrated that while weight teasing was a risk factor for eating disorder development in both obese and normal-weight children and adolescents, weight teasing was more commonly directed at overweight and obese individuals [72, 73]. This supports the idea that obesity is a risk factor for disordered eating, mediated by the stigma associated with obesity. Further evidence for this order of events can be seen in Decaluwé et al. (2003), who conducted a study of 196 patients at two pediatric weight-loss clinics. The study found that the age of onset of overweight/obesity preceded the age of onset of binge-eating behaviors [74]. Overly restrictive dieting behaviors and weight loss were also more prevalent in adolescents with a history of obesity, and individuals who were previously obese were often identified later in their disease course than their normal-weight counterparts [77]. This study by Lebow et al. (2015) highlights not only the role of obesity across the spectrum of eating disorders, but also the failure to recognize eating disorders in obese individuals, potentially because their weight loss, even if dramatic, was seen as a positive rather than an area of concern.

Given these intersections between obesity and eating disorders, some investigators and health care professionals have advocated for an integrated approach for interventions tackling obesity and eating disorders. There is a concern that the current language and methodology regarding weight loss for obese individuals may predispose them to excessive preoccupation with dietary habits, exercise, or body image [78, 79]. There are now some studies that evaluate integrated approaches that combine CBT for eating disorders with behavioral weight-loss therapy [80], but no definitive conclusions can be drawn yet regarding their efficacy.

Substance use disorder

In the adult population, obesity may actually be a protective factor for substance abuse, although the results from studies on the topic have been inconsistent [81]. Simon et al. (2006) conducted a cross-sectional study of 9125 US adults, reporting an odds ratio of 0.78 regarding the relationship between obesity and substance use disorders. Similar results were noted in a prospective cohort study by Pickering et al. (2011) using the US National Epidemiological Survey on Alcohol and Related Conditions (NESARC) [9]. However, this study did note an increased risk of alcohol use disorder for overweight men only. The increased odds ratio for overweight men and alcohol abuse was seen as well in a cross-sectional study on the NESARC cohort. However, this study failed to demonstrate an association between BMI and illicit drug use, which differed from the results of the Pickering et al. (2011) study [82]. The results of other large epidemiological studies in countries outside the United States have been similarly ambiguous, indicating that this is an area of research that definitely warrants further study [83].

Some studies have attempted to explain the potential preventative effects of obesity on substance abuse through hypothesizing that the cause of obesity is a form of food addiction [83]. Studies using the same NESARC cohort have found that a family history of alcohol addiction attenuated the increased odds ratio between obesity and alcohol abuse, leading to the conclusion that overeating and food addiction operate on the same neurologic reward pathways as other drugs of abuse [84, 85]. This is supported by additional studies that have demonstrated that increased BMI was correlated with decreased alcohol consumption, indicating that overeating competes with alcohol for the same brain reward centers and that it results in less-rewarding effects of alcohol in obese individuals [86].

References

[1] Simon GE, Von Korff M, Saunders K, et al. Association between obesity and psychiatric disorders in the US adult population. Arch Gen Psychiatry 2006;63(7):824–30.

[2] Halfon N, Larson K, Slusser W. Associations between obesity and comorbid mental health, developmental, and physical health conditions in a nationally representative sample of us children aged 10 to 17. Acad Pediatr 2013;13(1):6–13.

[3] Scott KM, Bruffaerts R, Simon GE, et al. Obesity and mental disorders in the general population: results from the world mental health surveys. Int J Obes (Lond) 2008;32(1):192–200.

[4] Kivimäki M, Lawlor DA, Singh-Manoux A, et al. Common mental disorder and obesity-insight from four repeat measures over 19 years: prospective Whitehall II cohort study. BMJ 2009;339(7726):902–5.

[5] Singh G, Jackson CA, Dobson A, Mishra GD. Bidirectional association between weight change and depression in mid-aged women: a population-based longitudinal study. Int J Obes (Lond) 2014;38(4):591–6.

[6] Pan A, Sun Q, Czernichow S, et al. Bidirectional association between depression and obesity in middle-aged and older women. Int J Obes (Lond) 2012;36(4):595–602.

[7] Pan A, Keum N, Okereke OI, et al. Bidirectional association between depression and metabolic syndrome: a systematic review and meta-analysis of epidemiological studies. Diabetes Care 2012;35(5):1171–80.

[8] Luppino FS, De Wit LM, Bouvy PF, et al. Overweight, obesity, and depression: a systematic review and meta-analysis of longitudinal studies. Arch Gen Psychiatry 2010;67(3):220–9.

[9] Pickering RP, Goldstein RB, Hasin DS, et al. Temporal relationships between overweight and obesity and DSM-IV substance use, mood, and anxiety disorders: results from a prospective study, the national epidemiologic survey on alcohol and related conditions. J Clin Psychiatry 2011;72(11):1494–502.

[10] Mannan M, Mamun A, Doi S, Clavarino A. Prospective associations between depression and obesity for adolescent males and females—a systematic review and meta-analysis of longitudinal studies. PLoS One 2016;11(6) e0157240.

[11] Hamer M, Batty GD, Kivimaki M. Risk of future depression in people who are obese but metabolically healthy: the English longitudinal study of ageing. Mol Psychiatry 2012;17 (9):940–5.
[12] Hryhorczuk C, Sharma S, Fulton SE. Metabolic disturbances connecting obesity and depression. Front Neurosci 2013;7:177.
[13] Amare AT, Schubert KO, Klingler-Hoffmann M, Cohen-Woods S, Baune BT. The genetic overlap between mood disorders and cardiometabolic diseases: a systematic review of genome wide and candidate gene studies. Transl Psychiatry 2017;7(1) e1007.
[14] Fuemmeler BF, Agurs-Collins T, McClernon FJ, Kollins SH, Garrett ME, Ashley-Koch AE. Interactions between genotype and depressive symptoms on obesity. Behav Genet 2009;39 (3):296–305.
[15] Milaneschi Y, Simonsick EM, Vogelzangs N, et al. Leptin, abdominal obesity, and onset of depression in older men and women. J Clin Psychiatry 2012;73(9):1205–11.
[16] Quteineh L, Preisig M, Rivera M, et al. Association of CRTC1 polymorphisms with obesity markers in subjects from the general population with lifetime depression. J Affect Disord 2016;198:43–9.
[17] Tyrrell J, Mulugeta A, Wood AR, et al. Using genetics to understand the causal influence of higher BMI on depression, Int J Epidemiol 2019;48(3):834–48. Available from: https://academic.oup.com/ije/article/48/3/834/5155677.
[18] Menzel JE, Schaefer LM, Burke NL, Mayhew LL, Brannick MT, Thompson JK. Appearance-related teasing, body dissatisfaction, and disordered eating: a meta-analysis. Body Image 2010;7(4):261–70.
[19] Weinberger NA, Kersting A, Riedel-Heller SG, Luck-Sikorski C. Body dissatisfaction in individuals with obesity compared to normal-weight individuals: a systematic review and meta-analysis, Obes Facts 2017;9(6):424–41. Available from: https://www.karger.com/Article/FullText/454837.
[20] Ferreiro F, Seoane G, Senra C. Toward understanding the role of body dissatisfaction in the gender differences in depressive symptoms and disordered eating: a longitudinal study during adolescence. J Adolesc 2014;37(1):73–84.
[21] Richard A, Rohrmann S, Lohse T, Eichholzer M. Is body weight dissatisfaction a predictor of depression independent of body mass index, sex and age? Results of a cross-sectional study. BMC Public Health 2016;16(1):863.
[22] de Wit LM, Fokkema M, van Straten A, Lamers F, Cuijpers P, BWJH P. Depressive and anxiety disorders and the association with obesity, physical, and social activities. Depress Anxiety 2010;27(11):1057–65. https://doi.org/10.1002/da.20738.
[23] Carroll DD, Blanck HM, Serdula MK, Brown DR. Obesity, physical activity, and depressive symptoms in a cohort of adults aged 51 to 61. J Aging Health 2010;22(3):384–98. Available from http://www.ncbi.nlm.nih.gov/pubmed/20164412.
[24] Vittengl JR. Mediation of the bidirectional relations between obesity and depression among women. Psychiatry Res 2018;264:254–9.
[25] Simon GE, Ludman EJ, Linde JA, et al. Association between obesity and depression in middle-aged women. Gen Hosp Psychiatry 2008;30(1):32–9.
[26] Danese A, Tan M. Childhood maltreatment and obesity: systematic review and meta-analysis. Mol Psychiatry 2014;19(5):544–54.
[27] Bentley T, Widom CS. A 30-year follow-up of the effects of child abuse and neglect on obesity in adulthood. Obesity 2009;17(10):1900–5. https://doi.org/10.1038/oby.2009.160.

[28] Shin SH, Miller DP. A longitudinal examination of childhood maltreatment and adolescent obesity: results from the National Longitudinal Study of Adolescent Health (AddHealth) Study. Child Abuse Negl 2012;36(2):84–94.
[29] Van Geel M, Vedder P, Tanilon J. Are overweight and obese youths more often bullied by their peers? A meta-analysis on the relation between weight status and bullying. Int J Obes (Lond) 2014;38(10):1263–7.
[30] Kukaswadia A, Craig W, Janssen I, Pickett W. Obesity as a determinant of two forms of bullying in ontario youth: a short report. Obes Facts 2011;4(6):469–72. Available from: https://www.karger.com/Article/FullText/335215.
[31] Griffiths LJ, Wolke D, Page AS, Horwood JP. Obesity and bullying: different effects for boys and girls. Arch Dis Child 2006;91(2):121–5.
[32] Bacchini D, Licenziati MR, Garrasi A, et al. Bullying and victimization in overweight and obese outpatient children and adolescents: an italian multicentric study. PLoS One 2015;10 (11) e0142715.
[33] Baldwin JR, Arseneault L, Odgers C, et al. Childhood bullying victimization and overweight in young adulthood: a cohort study. Psychosom Med 2016;78(9):1094–103.
[34] Mamun AA, O'Callaghan MJ, Williams GM, Najman JM. Adolescents bullying and young adults body mass index and obesity: a longitudinal study. Int J Obes (Lond) 2013;37 (8):1140–6.
[35] Takizawa R, Danese A, Maughan B, Arseneault L. Bullying victimization in childhood predicts inflammation and obesity at mid-life: a five-decade birth cohort study. Psychol Med 2015;45(13):2705–15.
[36] Sutin AR, Robinson E, Daly M, Terracciano A. Parent-reported bullying and child weight gain between ages 6 and 15. Child Obes 2016;12(6):482–7.
[37] Olvera N, Dempsey A, Gonzalez E, Abrahamson C. Weight-related teasing, emotional eating, and weight control behaviors in Hispanic and African American girls. Eat Behav 2013;14 (4):513–7.
[38] Lee KS, Vaillancourt T. Body mass index, peer victimization, and body dissatisfaction across 7 years of childhood and adolescence: evidence of moderated and mediated pathways. Dev Sci 2019;22(2) e12734.
[39] Brewerton TD, O'neil PM, Dansky BS, Kilpatrick DG. Extreme obesity and its associations with victimization, PTSD, major depression and eating disorders in a national sample of women. J Obes Eat Disord 2015;1(2). Available from: http://www.imedpub.com/http://obesity.imedpub.com/.
[40] Smith BN, Tyzik AL, Neylan TC, Cohen BE. PTSD and obesity in younger and older veterans: results from the mind your heart study. Psychiatry Res 2015;229(3):895–900.
[41] Dorflinger LM, Masheb RM. PTSD is associated with emotional eating among veterans seeking treatment for overweight/obesity. Eat Behav 2018;31:8–11.
[42] Kubzansky LD, Bordelois P, Jun HJ, et al. The weight of traumatic stress: a prospective study of posttraumatic stress disorder symptoms and weight status in women. JAMA Psychiat 2014;71(1):44–51.
[43] Farr OM, Sloan DM, Keane TM, Mantzoros CS. Stress- and PTSD-associated obesity and metabolic dysfunction: a growing problem requiring further research and novel treatments. Metabolism 2014;63(12):1463–8.
[44] Farhat T, Iannotti RJ, Simons-Morton BG. Overweight, obesity, youth, and health-risk behaviors. Am J Prev Med 2010;38(3):258–67.

[45] Gearhardt AN, Waller R, Jester JM, Hyde LW, Zucker RA. Body mass index across adolescence and substance use problems in early adulthood. Psychol Addict Behav 2018;32(3):309–19. https://doi.org/10.1037/adb0000365.supp.
[46] Laxer RE, Brownson RC, Dubin JA, Cooke M, Chaurasia A, Leatherdale ST. Clustering of risk-related modifiable behaviours and their association with overweight and obesity among a large sample of youth in the COMPASS study. BMC Public Health 2017;17(1):102.
[47] Huang DYC, Lanza HI, Anglin MD. Association between adolescent substance use and obesity in young adulthood: a group-based dual trajectory analysis. Addict Behav 2013;38(11):2653–60.
[48] Huang DYC, Lanza HI, Wright-Volel K, Anglin MD. Developmental trajectories of childhood obesity and risk behaviors in adolescence. J Adolesc 2013;36(1):139–48.
[49] Lanza HI, Grella CE, Chung PJ. Adolescent obesity and future substance use: incorporating the psychosocial context. J Adolesc 2015;45:20–30.
[50] Lanza HI, Grella CE, Chung PJ. Does adolescent weight status predict problematic substance use patterns? Am J Health Behav 2014;38(5):708–16.
[51] Pasch KE, Velazquez CE, Cance JD, Moe SG, Lytle LA. Youth substance use and body composition: does risk in one area predict risk in the other? J Youth Adolesc 2012;41(1):14–26.
[52] Zuba A, Warschburger P. The role of weight teasing and weight bias internalization in psychological functioning: a prospective study among school-aged children. Eur Child Adolesc Psychiatry 2017;26(10):1245–55.
[53] Cortese S, Moreira-Maia CR, St Fleur D, Morcillo-Peñalver C, Rohde LA, Faraone SV. Association between ADHD and obesity: a systematic review and meta-analysis. Am J Psychiatry 2016;173(1):34–43.
[54] Nigg JT, Johnstone JM, Musser ED, Long HG, Willoughby M, Shannon J. Attention-deficit/hyperactivity disorder (ADHD) and being overweight/obesity: new data and meta-analysis. Clin Psychol Rev 2016;43:67–79.
[55] Khalife N, Kantomaa M, Glover V, et al. Childhood attention-deficit/hyperactivity disorder symptoms are risk factors for obesity and physical inactivity in adolescence. J Am Acad Child Adolesc Psychiatry 2014;53(4):425–36.
[56] Cortese S, Ramos Olazagasti MA, Klein RG, Castellanos FX, Proal E, Mannuzza S. Obesity in men with childhood ADHD: a 33-year controlled, prospective, follow-up study. Pediatrics 2013;131(6) e1731-8.
[57] Aguirre Castaneda RL, Kumar S, Voigt RG, et al. Childhood attention-deficit/hyperactivity disorder, sex, and obesity: a longitudinal population-based study. Mayo Clin Proc 2016;91(3):352–61.
[58] Cortese S. The association between ADHD and obesity: intriguing, progressively more investigated, but still puzzling. Brain Sci 2019;9(10).
[59] Taylor VH, Forhan M, Vigod SN, McIntyre RS, Morrison KM. The impact of obesity on quality of life. Best Pract Res Clin Endocrinol Metab 2013;27(2):139–46.
[60] Puhl RM, King KM. Weight discrimination and bullying. Best Pract Res Clin Endocrinol Metab 2013;27(2):117–27. https://doi.org/10.1016/j.beem.2012.12.002.
[61] O'Brien KS, Latner JD, Ebneter D, Hunter JA. Obesity discrimination: the role of physical appearance, personal ideology, and anti-fat prejudice. Int J Obes (Lond) 2013;37(3):455–60.
[62] Giel KE, Zipfel S, Alizadeh M, et al. Stigmatization of obese individuals by human resource professionals: an experimental study. BMC Public Health 2012;12(1) 525.
[63] Phelan SM, Burgess DJ, Yeazel MW, Hellerstedt WL, Griffin JM, van Ryn M. Impact of weight bias and stigma on quality of care and outcomes for patients with obesity. Obes Rev 2015;16(4):319–26. https://doi.org/10.1111/obr.12266.

[64] Tomiyama AJ, Carr D, Granberg EM, et al. How and why weight stigma drives the obesity 'epidemic' and harms health. BMC Med 2018;16(1):123. https://doi.org/10.1186/s12916-018-1116-5.

[65] Ali MM, Rizzo JA, Heiland FW. Big and beautiful? Evidence of racial differences in the perceived attractiveness of obese females. J Adolesc 2013;36(3):539–49.

[66] Lieberman DL, Tybur JM, Latner JD. Disgust sensitivity, obesity stigma, and gender: contamination psychology predicts weight bias for women, not men. Obesity 2012;20(9):1803–14. https://doi.org/10.1038/oby.2011.247.

[67] Boyes AD, Latner JD. Weight stigma in existing romantic relationships. J Sex Marital Ther 2009;35(4):282–93. https://doi.org/10.1080/00926230902851280.

[68] Lewer M, Bauer A, Hartmann AS, Vocks S. Different facets of body image disturbance in binge eating disorder: a review. Nutrients 2017;9(12).

[69] Darby A, Hay P, Mond J, Quirk F, Buttner P, Kennedy L. The rising prevalence of comorbid obesity and eating disorder behaviors from 1995 to 2005. Int J Eat Disord 2009;42(2):104–8. https://doi.org/10.1002/eat.20601.

[70] Da Luz FQ, Sainsbury A, Mannan H, Touyz S, Mitchison D, Hay P. Prevalence of obesity and comorbid eating disorder behaviors in South Australia from 1995 to 2015. Int J Obes (Lond) 2017;41(7):1148–53.

[71] Burrows A, Cooper M. Possible risk factors in the development of eating disorders in overweight pre-adolescent girls. Int J Obes (Lond) 2002;26(9):1268–73.

[72] Neumark-Sztainer D, Falkner N, Story M, Perry C, Hannan PJ, Mulert S. Weight-teasing among adolescents: correlations with weight status and disordered eating behaviors. Int J Obes (Lond) 2002;26(1):123–31.

[73] Fitzpatrick E, Dew TK, Quaglia A, Sherwood RA, Mitry RR, Dhawan A. Analysis of adipokine concentrations in paediatric non-alcoholic fatty liver disease. Pediatr Obes 2012;7 (6):471–9. https://doi.org/10.1111/j.2047-6310.2012.00078.x.

[74] Decaluwé V, Braet C. Prevalence of binge-eating disorder in obese children and adolescents seeking weight-loss treatment. Int J Obes (Lond) 2003;27(3):404–9.

[75] Haines J, Neumark-Sztainer D. Prevention of obesity and eating disorders: a consideration of shared risk factors. Health Educ Res 2006;21(6):770–82.

[76] Neumark-Sztainer DR, Wall MM, Haines JI, Story MT, Sherwood NE, van den Berg PA. Shared risk and protective factors for overweight and disordered eating in adolescents. Am J Prev Med 2007;33(5):359–69.

[77] Lebow J, Sim LA, Kransdorf LN. Prevalence of a history of overweight and obesity in adolescents with restrictive eating disorders. J Adolesc Health 2015;56(1):19–24.

[78] Golden NH, Schneider M, Wood C, et al. Preventing obesity and eating disorders in adolescents. Pediatrics 2016;138(3).

[79] da Luz FQ, Hay P, Touyz S, Sainsbury A. Obesity with comorbid eating disorders: associated health risks and treatment approaches. Nutrients 2018;10(7).

[80] da Luz FQ, Swinbourne J, Sainsbury A, et al. HAPIFED: a healthy approach to weight management and food in eating disorders: a case series and manual development. J Eat Disord 2017;5(1).

[81] Amiri S, Behnezhad S. Obesity and substance use: a systematic review and meta-analysis. Obes Med 2018;11:31–41.

[82] Barry D, Petry NM. Associations between body mass index and substance use disorders differ by gender: results from the National Epidemiologic Survey on alcohol and related conditions. Addict Behav 2009;34(1):51–60.

[83] Sansone RA, Sansone LA. Obesity and substance misuse: is there a relationship? Innov Clin Neurosci 2013;10(9–10):30–5.

[84] Gearhardt AN, Corbin WR. Body mass index and alcohol consumption: family history of alcoholism as a moderator. Psychol Addict Behav 2009;23(2):216–25.

[85] Grucza RA, Krueger RF, Racette SB, Norberg KE, Hipp PR, Bierut LJ. The emerging link between alcoholism risk and obesity in the United States. Arch Gen Psychiatry 2010;67 (12):1301–8.

[86] Kleiner KD, Gold MS, Frost-Pineda K, Lenz-Brunsman B, Perri MG, Jacobs WS. Body mass index and alcohol use. J Addict Dis 2004;23(3):105–18.

Chapter 8

The role of diet in the obesity epidemic

Elizabeth Kiwanuka, M.D., Ph.D.
Department of Plastic Surgery, Rhode Island Hospital, Providence, RI, United States

Introduction

Studies have shown that food consumption increases when more food is available [1]. Over the past decades, per capita, US food availability has increased by three-fold; however, the way our diet affects our energy balance is complex [2]. Daily energy expenditure depends on total energy intake (kilocalories consumed), macronutrient composition (fat, protein, and carbohydrates), the energy density of the food (kilocalories per gram of food), and the timing of the food intake. Besides, economic and policy influences to maximize food production have to build industrialized systems that produce and market highly processed foods rich in corn, soy, sugars, etc. [3]. The unnaturally high amounts of salt, sugar, fat, and flavor additives increase consumption. Also, changes in behavior and lifestyle with snacking between meals and more people eating in restaurants likely lead to increased calorie intake, thereby causing obesity [4, 5].

Obesity is a state of increased body weight, characterized by an increased number and size of adipocytes [6]. The stage of triglycerides in adipose tissue is determined by the interaction between genetic, environmental, and psychosocial factors. Although the role of genes in obesity is well established, one can assume that the rising prevalence of obesity has not been due to a recent change in genetics [7]. Besides, the control of food intake has a more significant influence on energy balance than small changes in metabolic rates. A modest imbalance between energy intake and energy expenditure may result in severe obesity over time; a daily energy intake that exceeds expenditure by 5% leads to a 5-kg weight gain over 1 year. Daily variations of food intake have a coefficient of $\pm 23\%$, whereas daily fluctuations in energy expenditure are $\pm 2\%$, indicating that food intake is the most important determinant. This chapter reviews the role of diet in the development of obesity.

Obesity. https://doi.org/10.1016/B978-0-12-818839-2.00008-9

The energy balance equation

Weight gain is often a consequence of sustained periods of excess calorie intake while body weight is a function of genetic, environmental, and psychosocial factors. These factors ultimately lead to a chronic alteration of the energy balance equation:

$$\text{Energy intake} > \text{energy expenditure} => \text{weight gain}$$

This approach is based on fundamental thermodynamic principles by Hess and Helmholtz that energy cannot be destroyed and can only be gained, lost, or stored by an organism. The concept of energy balance is fundamental to obesity treatment with dietary management. It is focusing on reducing energy intake while holding energy expenditure consent—targeting voluntary behaviors. Pharmaceutical management, in contrast, targets the metabolism by blocking the absorption of nutrients or affecting signals of appetite or satiety while surgical management modifies the anatomy and thereby limits the capacity for energy absorption, bypassing voluntary behaviors [8].

The energy balance has many limitations for explaining obesity in humans and simplifies the complexity of energy balance in humans [9]. If energy intake exceeds energy expenditure, increased body weight should lead to a result in higher energy expenditure, eventually reaching a new plateau. Thermodynamic theory is well established; however, it may not fully explain the dynamic process as many biological and compensational mechanisms respond to periods of energy deficiency or surfeit.

Appetite regulation

Appetite regulation plays a major role in the etiology of obesity [10, 11]. Our daily food intake depends on both homeostatic (e.g., energy needs) and nonhomeostatic (e.g., environmental factors, habits) [12]. These complex processes involve psychological and behavioral patterns as well as peripheral physiological and metabolic mechanisms. The suppression of hunger at the end of a meal is called satiation while satiety is the period of absence of hunger between meals [13].

Recent evidence suggests that the volume of food plays a major role in eliciting satiation and satiety. The gastrointestinal tract contains mechanoreceptors that are stimulated by bulk. There are also chemoreceptors that detect the nature of nutrients digested. These receptors relay the information to the brain via the vagus nerve and can induce both satiation and early satiety [14, 15].

Leptin is a hormone secreted by adipocytes and influences food intake by acting on the hypothalamus [16]. Leptin is secreted in proportion to adipose tissue mass. In mice, leptin inhibits feeding and stimulates energy expenditure. In obese humans, although plasma leptin concentrations correlate to the mass of the adipose tissue, they do not induce a reduction in food intake and an increase in energy expenditure. These findings suggest that obese humans have developed resistance to leptin. By contrast, leptin promotes the maintenance of adequate energy stores, likely for survival during periods of starvation. During periods of fasting, reduced leptin levels tend to limit weight loss by stimulating hunger and the suppression of plasma thyroid hormone levels [17–19].

The effect of macronutrients on obesity

The macronutrient composition of food influences satiety and appetite [20]. The body's ability to utilize different nutrients is inversely related to the cost of absorbing, processing, and storing the nutrient. This process, known as thermogenesis, reflects the differences in energy cost for synthesis for fat, proteins, and carbohydrates, respectively. The thermogenic effect of lipids is 2–3%, which gives an energy efficiency of 97–98%. Proteins have a thermic effect of 25–30%, and carbohydrates have 6–8% (Table 1) [21].

The type of food we consume in Western diets has shifted from whole grains, vegetables, and legumes to carbohydrates that are digested rapidly, resulting in a high glycemic load and increased insulin demand [22, 23]. Meals with high-fat content easily lead to overconsumption, and the high energy density of fatty meals promotes higher energy intake. Passive overconsumption of food seems to correlate to energy density. This is likely because people tend to consume a similar bulk of food regardless of its composition. Moreover, alcohol is often additive to the Western diet and may represent as much as 5–10% of the energy intake [24]. Alcohol is oxidized in competition to fats and that in combination with the energy of alcohol contributes to weight gain [25, 26].

Carbohydrates

Adults are recommended to get 45–65% of their daily calories from carbohydrates. Carbohydrates have a relatively low energy density (4 kcal per gram as compared to 9 kcal per gram of fat), and a high carbohydrate diet is bulkier and more filling. After a meal, glucose leads to an increase in plasma insulin, and the insulin subsequently promotes glucose uptake and oxidation in insulin-sensitive

TABLE 1 Energy and macronutrients.

	Fat	Protein	Carbohydrate
kcal per g	9	4	4
Thermogenesis	Low	High	Medium
Satiating capacity	Low	High	Medium

tissues. Moreover, insulin suppresses the activity of hormone-sensitive lipase and thereby inhibits lipolysis and lipid oxidation. Thus, a meal rich in carbohydrates stimulates insulin secretion and glucose oxidation while inhibiting fat oxidation [27].

Dietary carbohydrates may also indirectly play a role in weight gain by stimulating de novo lipogenesis (fat tissue transformation) [28, 29]. But even in situations with massive carbohydrate overfeeding, de novo lipogenesis does not exceed 3–10 g of fatty acids synthesized per day, thus it does not contribute significantly to body fat stores [30].

High-fructose corn syrup has been identified as an independent risk factor for obesity. Fructose is typically derived from sucrose, high-fructose corn syrup, or fruit. Table sugar contains 50% glucose and 50% fructose, honey 38% fructose, and agave 90% fructose. Fructose adds calories and does not affect the appetite control system. In addition, fructose has also been linked to central adiposity, gout, and hyperlipidemia [31].

Fat

The recommended daily dietary intake of fat in adults is 20–30% of the total calorie intake. Dietary fat contains 9 kcal per gram, twice the energy density of proteins and carbohydrates. Dietary fat has a low thermic effect and is less satiating than other macronutrients. Consuming fat leads to accumulation in the body fat because fat does not promote its oxidation. After fatty meals, lipid oxidation is not stimulated, and the dietary fat consumed is primarily deposited in adipose tissue [32]. So when the energy balance is positive, the fat is stored in the adipose tissue. In contrast, when the energy balance is negative, the endogenous lipids are oxidized to make up for the deficit. Therefore, in the past, reducing fat intake was the primary focus of dietary prevention [8, 33].

The notion that dietary fat is the primary driver of obesity was supported by studies showing that ad libitum low-fat diets result on average in a 3–4 kg weight loss. However, unfortunately, the weigh is frequently regained after cessation of the diet. Furthermore, the low-fat diets that were popular during the 1980s and 1990s did not successfully slow down the obesity epidemic [34, 35].

Proteins

The body's protein balance is highly regulated [36]. The recommended dietary allowance for protein is between 0.8 and 1 g per kilogram of body weight, and an intake of protein beyond the requirements only causes a transient positive nitrogen balance. Despite that, high-protein diets have become popular [37]. Protein is the most satiating macronutrient, and high-protein diets are believed to suppress hunger to a greater extent than fat and carbohydrates. Furthermore, the more significant thermogenic effect of proteins contributes to the reduced calorie intake [36].

High-fat and high-protein diets both aim to reduce insulin secretion [38]. As discussed above, carbohydrates are the primary stimulant of insulin release, and high protein diets do not stimulate insulin release, thereby promoting fat oxidation. Several studies have also found more significant fat loss with high-protein diets despite similar weight loss [39, 40].

Obesity and diets

Hypocaloric diets

A modest weight loss of 0.5 kg per week can be achieved by reducing the daily energy intake by 500 kcal [41]. Traditional hypocaloric diets aim at reducing daily energy intake by 250–500 kcal, leading to a daily intake of 1200–1500 kcal for women and 1500–1800 kcal for men [42].

In order to restrict caloric intake, these diets tend to contain 30% fat, 50% carbohydrate, and 20% protein. The weight loss is typically seen in the first month before slowing down because of hormonal adaptation, preventing further weight loss. Hypocaloric diets are effective for short-term weight loss, but long-term adherence to these diets is challenging to accomplish [43–45].

Intermittent energy restriction

Intermittent energy restriction diets have gained popularity and are based on periods of reduced energy intake alternated with unrestricted feeding [46–48]. The schedules vary and include alternate day fasting or 5:2 diet regimens. The restricted diet often allows about 500 kcal. No studies have shown that intermittent diets can prevent weight gain in normal-weight individuals, and there is limited data on the efficiency of intermittent dieting on weight loss. Some studies in animal models and normal-weight humans have raised safety concerns as they show that intermittent diets alter the metabolic hemostasis.

The optimal pattern of energy restriction remains controversial, and it is unclear which macronutrient is the optimal composition of such intermittent diets [49–51].

Plant-based diet

The Academy of Nutrition and Dietetics position paper states that vegan and vegetarian diets "are healthful, nutritionally adequate, and may provide health benefits in the prevention and treatment of certain diseases." The term plant-based diet includes vegan and vegetarian diets and is based around fruits, vegetables, grains, and legumes. The vegetarian diet typically also includes dairy products as well as eggs. Plant-based diets are beneficial for several health conditions such as cardiovascular, blood pressure, and diabetes. Moreover, plant-based diets have been proposed to reduce obesity-induced chronic inflammation, and thereby prevent the chronic disease risk associated with obesity [52, 53].

Interestingly, plant-based diets have been associated with weight loss, and in observational studies, people who follow plant-based diets typically have lower body weights compared to other individuals. The inverse association between plant-based diets and obesity has several explanations. Plant-based diets are rich in fiber, chlorogenic acids, antioxidants, and plant protein. These components can modify things such as satiety, inflammation, oxidative stress, and gut microbiome composition. Besides, the high-fiber content reduces the energy density of the meal. Moreover, plant-based diets are low in fat, which has been suggested to be beneficial for the prevention of obesity [54, 55].

Fast food and trans fatty acids

Fast food is mass-produced food that is made for commercial resale and prioritizes "speed of service." Fast-food consumption has increased drastically in the United States as well as worldwide in the past decade, now accounting for as much as 10% of total energy intake per person [56]. Many studies have shown a strong correlation between fast food intake and weight gain and the consumption of fast food is also associated with the development of insulin resistance [57, 58].

There are many ways that fast-food consumption can lead to weight gain and obesity-associated health problems [59]. Fast food has a high caloric density, so the total caloric content of a meal is often higher than a home-cooked meal. Fast food also has a high content of industrially produced trans fatty acids because they have higher melting points, better taste, and longer shelf lives compared to other fats [60, 61]. A daily intake of 5 g of trans fat is associated with a 25% increase in the risk of ischemic heart disease [62]. Trans fatty acids produce a unique cardiometabolic imprint and have been linked to insulin-resistance syndrome [63–65]. Trans fatty acids are industrially produced and not naturally present in foods, and should be considered a food additive with health value but significant potential for harm [66].

References

[1] Vandevijvere S, et al. Increased food energy supply as a major driver of the obesity epidemic: a global analysis. Bull World Health Organ 2015;93(7):446–56.

[2] Hall KD, Guo J. Obesity energetics: body weight regulation and the effects of diet composition. Gastroenterology 2017;152(7):1718–1727. e3.

[3] Ogden CL, et al. The epidemiology of obesity. Gastroenterology 2007;132(6):2087–102.

[4] Swinburn BA, et al. The global obesity pandemic: shaped by global drivers and local environments. Lancet 2011;378(9793):804–14.

[5] Hall KD, et al. The progressive increase of food waste in America and its environmental impact. PLoS One 2009;4(11). e7940.

[6] Engin A. The definition and prevalence of obesity and metabolic syndrome. Adv Exp Med Biol 2017;960:1–17.

[7] Crujeiras AB, et al. Leptin resistance in obesity: an epigenetic landscape. Life Sci 2015;140:57–63.

[8] Jequier E. Pathways to obesity. Int J Obes Relat Metab Disord 2002;26(Suppl 2):S12–7.

[9] Livingston EH, Kohlstadt I. Simplified resting metabolic rate-predicting formulas for normal-sized and obese individuals. Obes Res 2005;13(7):1255–62.

[10] Strain GW, Hershcopf RJ, Zumoff B. Food intake of very obese persons: quantitative and qualitative aspects. J Am Diet Assoc 1992;92(2):199–203.

[11] Blundell JE, Gillett A. Control of food intake in the obese. Obes Res 2001;9(Suppl. 4): 263s–70s.

[12] Turner A, et al. Interactions between bitter taste, diet and dysbiosis: consequences for appetite and obesity. Nutrients 2018;10(10).

[13] Hopkins M, Blundell JE. Energy balance, body composition, sedentariness and appetite regulation: pathways to obesity. Clin Sci (Lond) 2016;130(18):1615–28.

[14] Valassi E, Scacchi M, Cavagnini F. Neuroendocrine control of food intake. Nutr Metab Cardiovasc Dis 2008;18(2):158–68.

[15] Babcock Gilbert S, Roth LW. Hypothalamic obesity. Minerva Endocrinol 2015;40(1):61–70.

[16] Jung CH, Kim MS. Molecular mechanisms of central leptin resistance in obesity. Arch Pharm Res 2013;36(2):201–7.

[17] Mechanick JI, Zhao S, Garvey WT. Leptin, an adipokine with central importance in the global obesity problem. Glob Heart 2018;13(2):113–27.

[18] Stubbs RJ. Nutrition society medal lecture. Appetite, feeding behaviour and energy balance in human subjects. Proc Nutr Soc 1998;57(3):341–56.

[19] Gasque G. An appetite for understanding appetite. PLoS Biol 2017;15(5). e2002838.

[20] Astrup A, Raben A. Obesity: an inherited metabolic deficiency in the control of macronutrient balance? Eur J Clin Nutr 1992;46(9):611–20.

[21] Bray GA, Siri-Tarino PW. The role of macronutrient content in the diet for weight management. Endocrinol Metab Clin North Am 2016;45(3):581–604.

[22] Astrup A. Dietary composition, substrate balances and body fat in subjects with a predisposition to obesity. Int J Obes Relat Metab Disord 1993;17(Suppl. 3):S32–6, discussion S41–S42.

[23] Romaguera D, et al. Food composition of the diet in relation to changes in waist circumference adjusted for body mass index. PLoS One 2011;6(8). e23384.

[24] Flatt JP. Body weight, fat storage, and alcohol metabolism. Nutr Rev 1992;50(9):267–70.

[25] Traversy G, Chaput JP. Alcohol consumption and obesity: an update. Curr Obes Rep 2015; 4(1):122–30.

[26] Brandhagen M, et al. Alcohol and macronutrient intake patterns are related to general and central adiposity. Eur J Clin Nutr 2012;66(3):305–13.

[27] Sartorius K, et al. Does high-carbohydrate intake lead to increased risk of obesity? A systematic review and meta-analysis. BMJ Open 2018;8(2). e018449.

[28] Hall KD. A review of the carbohydrate–insulin model of obesity. Eur J Clin Nutr 2017;71(3): 323–6.

[29] Madsen L, et al. Dietary proteins, brown fat, and adiposity. Front Physiol 2018;9:1792.

[30] van Dam RM, Seidell JC. Carbohydrate intake and obesity. Eur J Clin Nutr 2007;61(Suppl 1): S75–99.

[31] Aarsland A, Chinkes D, Wolfe RR. Hepatic and whole-body fat synthesis in humans during carbohydrate overfeeding. Am J Clin Nutr 1997;65(6):1774–82.

[32] Astrup A. The role of dietary fat in obesity. Semin Vasc Med 2005;5(1):40–7.

[33] Flatt JP. Macronutrient composition and food selection. Obes Res 2001;9(Suppl. 4): 256s–262s.
[34] Golay A, Bobbioni E. The role of dietary fat in obesity. Int J Obes Relat Metab Disord 1997;21 (Suppl 3):S2–11.
[35] Astrup A. The role of dietary fat in the prevention and treatment of obesity. Efficacy and safety of low-fat diets. Int J Obes Relat Metab Disord 2001;25(Suppl. 1):S46–50.
[36] Westerterp-Plantenga MS. Protein intake and energy balance. Regul Pept 2008;149(1–3): 67–9.
[37] Simpson SJ, Raubenheimer D. Obesity: the protein leverage hypothesis. Obes Rev 2005;6(2): 133–42.
[38] Promintzer M, Krebs M. Effects of dietary protein on glucose homeostasis. Curr Opin Clin Nutr Metab Care 2006;9(4):463–8.
[39] Martens EA, Lemmens SG, Westerterp-Plantenga MS. Protein leverage affects energy intake of high-protein diets in humans. Am J Clin Nutr 2012;97(1):86–93.
[40] Martens EA, et al. Protein leverage effects of beef protein on energy intake in humans. Am J Clin Nutr 2014;99(6):1397–406.
[41] Koliaki C, et al. Defining the optimal dietary approach for safe, effective and sustainable weight loss in overweight and obese adults. Healthcare (Basel) 2018;6(3).
[42] Finer N. Low-calorie diets and sustained weight loss. Obes Res 2001;9(Suppl 4):290s–4s.
[43] Wilkinson DL, McCargar L. Is there an optimal macronutrient mix for weight loss and weight maintenance? Best Pract Res Clin Gastroenterol 2004;18(6):1031–47.
[44] Malik VS, Hu FB. Popular weight-loss diets: from evidence to practice. Nat Clin Pract Cardiovasc Med 2007;4(1):34–41.
[45] Johnstone A. Fasting for weight loss: an effective strategy or latest dieting trend? Int J Obes (Lond) 2015;39(5):727–33.
[46] Aksungar FB, et al. Comparison of intermittent fasting versus caloric restriction in obese subjects: a two year follow-up. J Nutr Health Aging 2017;21(6):681–5.
[47] Gotthardt JD, Bello NT. Meal pattern alterations associated with intermittent fasting for weight loss are normalized after high-fat diet re-feeding. Physiol Behav 2017;174:49–56.
[48] Mattson MP, Longo VD, Harvie M. Impact of intermittent fasting on health and disease processes. Ageing Res Rev 2017;39:46–58.
[49] Antoni R, et al. Effects of intermittent fasting on glucose and lipid metabolism. Proc Nutr Soc 2017;76(3):361–8.
[50] Harvie M, Howell A. Potential Benefits and harms of intermittent energy restriction and intermittent fasting amongst obese, overweight and normal weight subjects—a narrative review of human and animal evidence. Behav Sci (Basel) 2017;7(1).
[51] Antoni R, et al. Intermittent v. continuous energy restriction: differential effects on postprandial glucose and lipid metabolism following matched weight loss in overweight/obese participants. Br J Nutr 2018;119(5):507–16.
[52] Barnard ND, Levin SM, Yokoyama Y. A systematic review and meta-analysis of changes in body weight in clinical trials of vegetarian diets. J Acad Nutr Diet 2015;115(6):954–69.
[53] Yokoyama Y, Levin SM, Barnard ND. Association between plant-based diets and plasma lipids: a systematic review and meta-analysis. Nutr Rev 2017;75(9):683–98.
[54] Satija A, et al. Plant-based dietary patterns and incidence of type 2 diabetes in US men and women: results from three prospective cohort studies. PLoS Med 2016;13(6). e1002039.
[55] Chen Z, et al. Plant-based diet and adiposity over time in a middle-aged and elderly population: the Rotterdam study. Epidemiology 2019;30(2):303–10.

[56] Paeratakul S, et al. Fast-food consumption among US adults and children: dietary and nutrient intake profile. J Am Diet Assoc 2003;103(10):1332–8.

[57] Wilcox S, et al. Frequency of consumption at fast-food restaurants is associated with dietary intake in overweight and obese women recruited from financially disadvantaged neighborhoods. Nutr Res 2013;33(8):636–46.

[58] Nguyen BT, Powell LM. The impact of restaurant consumption among US adults: effects on energy and nutrient intakes. Public Health Nutr 2014;17(11):2445–52.

[59] Mohammadbeigi A, et al. Fast food consumption and overweight/obesity prevalence in students and its association with general and abdominal obesity. J Prev Med Hyg 2018;59(3): E236–40.

[60] Wang Y, Proctor SD. Current issues surrounding the definition of trans-fatty acids: implications for health, industry and food labels. Br J Nutr 2013;110(8):1369–83.

[61] Hansen CP, et al. Adipose tissue trans-fatty acids and changes in body weight and waist circumference. Br J Nutr 2014;111(7):1283–91.

[62] Mozaffarian D, Willett WC. Trans fatty acids and cardiovascular risk: a unique cardiometabolic imprint? Curr Atheroscler Rep 2007;9(6):486–93.

[63] Micha R, Mozaffarian D. Trans fatty acids: effects on cardiometabolic health and implications for policy. Prostaglandins Leukot Essent Fatty Acids 2008;79(3–5):147–52.

[64] Mozaffarian D, Aro A, Willett WC. Health effects of trans-fatty acids: experimental and observational evidence. Eur J Clin Nutr 2009;63(Suppl 2):S5–21.

[65] Nestel P. Trans fatty acids: are its cardiovascular risks fully appreciated? Clin Ther 2014;36(3): 315–21.

[66] Ginter E, Simko V. New data on harmful effects of trans-fatty acids. Bratisl Lek Listy 2016;117(5):251–3.

Chapter 9

The role of physical activity in the obesity epidemic

Elizabeth Kiwanuka, M.D., Ph.D.
Department of Plastic Surgery, Rhode Island Hospital, Providence, RI, United States

Introduction

Overweight and obesity are significant public health concerns and are associated with numerous health problems, including diabetes, cardiovascular disease, musculoskeletal disorders, and some forms of cancer [1, 2]. Obesity develops when calories consumed exceed energy expenditure, but the disease process is complex and different genetic and environmental factors contribute [3–8].

Body weight is regulated by the energy equation where the energy balance is the sum of the calories consumed minus the calories expended. Therefore, when energy intake is equal to energy expenditure, the body weight remains stable [9]. Studies have shown that the most effective way to achieve a negative energy balance is a combination of exercise and diet [10]. Creating a negative energy balance by decreasing energy intake or increasing energy expenditure though exercise is a common strategy for weight loss. Weight management depends on dietary modifications and energy expenditure, and physical activity is the most variable component of energy expenditure. In addition, physical activity is important to long-term weight control and overall health by optimizing body composition and enhancing metabolic fitness. This chapter reviews the role of physical activity in the development of obesity.

Health benefits of physical activity

For general health benefits, exercising 3 days per week will lead to changes, but more frequent sessions will be more effective. The health-related benefits of physical activity include cardiorespiratory, endurance, muscular strength and endurance, flexibility, and body composition. These benefits occur in a dose-related manner with activity ranging from 15 to 100 min of exercise per day, leading to an all-cause mortality reduction by about 4% [11]. All levels of

Obesity. https://doi.org/10.1016/B978-0-12-818839-2.00009-0

physical activity are associated with reduced mortality when compared with insufficiently active individuals, and the health benefits are also seen in people with diabetes, hypertension, and metabolic syndrome as well as smokers.

Regular physical activity, such as aerobic or muscle-strengthening exercise, leads to adaptations in multiple body systems [12]. Aerobic exercise improves cardiorespiratory fitness, and resistance training increases muscle strength. Physical activity improves bone health, and regular aerobic or resistance exercise can reduce systolic blood. In addition, exercise leads to better cognitive function and can help with depression and anxiety.

Exercise and weight gain prevention

Because of the impact on energy balance, physical activity can contribute to the prevention of weight gain [13]. Data from observational studies have shown that regular exercise can prevent weight gain, and studies demonstrate an inverse association between measures of adiposity and physical activity [8, 14]. The National Health and Nutrition Examination Survey identified that low levels of self-reported physical activity are associated with a three-fold higher risk of significant weight gain in men, and that number is almost four-fold in women [15–17].

Exercise increases energy expenditure by altering physiological processes and affecting cellular mechanisms that accelerate the breakdown of the body's primary energy stores. Weight gain prevention is primarily achieved by the increase of glycogenolysis and fatty acid oxidation in muscle and liver as well as glycolysis, the citric acid cycle, and oxidative phosphorylation in muscles and lipolysis in adipose tissue and muscle [18].

The likelihood of maintaining a BMI of 18.5–25 kg per m^2 is increased when exercising approximately 167 min per week. Other studies have shown that vigorous-intensity physical activity of at least 1 h per week leads to a significant decrease in the incidence of obesity. Also, the odds were reduced in a dose–response manner relative to the level of physical activity [19]. The American College of Sports Medicine position stand also supported that physical activity prevent weight gain with 150–250 min per week of physical activity. This correlates to an approximate energy expenditure of 1200–2000 kcal per week [20].

Physical activity and weight loss

During active weight loss, the basal metabolic rate falls, making the physical activity even more important [21]. The American College of Sports Medicine, the European College of Sport Science, the American College of Cardiology, and the American Heart Association task force recommend 150 min of moderate-intensity exercise per week [20, 22–24]. This amount of exercise will, without dietary restrictions, induce a weight loss of about 2–3 kg. To achieve a clinically significant weight loss of 5%, the time of exercise increases to 225 to

420 min per week. It is estimated that every 50 min of exercise per week results in a loss of about 1 kg over 6 months [25, 26].

Clinical trials involving physical activity show numerous health benefits for overweight and obese individuals such as improved glucose control, endothelial function, lipid profile, and quality of life [27–33]. The type of exercise depends on the individual's needs and abilities. All physical activity will increase the energy expenditure, and as long as the total workload is the same, the modality does not significantly affect the outcome [34, 35]. All types of physical activity will reduce body mass as long as the energy expenditure exceeds energy intake. However, in the obese population, walking has proven to be the most effective mode of exercise because it has a low injury risk. Data suggest that a 1-h walk per day is the best exercise prescription for most obese individuals. Swimming is also an activity that helps reduce the loading on joints and thereby also the risk of injury. Importantly, resistance weight training helps maintain metabolically active tissue and is an essential component in the exercise prescription [36].

Programs consistent with public health recommendations lead to limited weight loss. The Dose Response to Exercise in Women study did not show a significant change in body weight in postmenopausal women exercising at public health guidelines for 6 months [33]. Similarly, the Inflammation and Exercise Study did not demonstrate a significant change in body weight compared to the control group after 4 months [37].

A sedentary lifestyle has been linked to the development of obesity, and the number of steps taken each day is often used as a marker [38–40]. A sedentary lifestyle is defined as <5000 steps per day, whereas an active lifestyle is >8000–10,000 steps per day. This is often measured using pedometers. Pedometer-based interventions where sedentary participants increase their physical activity by 2000–4000 steps per day showed an average weight loss of <2 kg [41, 42]. A metaanalysis by Richardson et al. on pedometer-based interventions without caloric restriction observed that the pooled estimated change in weight was 1.3 kg weight loss [43]. Bravata et al. performed a metaanalysis regarding the physiological effects of pedometer-based interventions and reported reductions in BMI of 0.38 kg per m^2 [44].

Clinically significant weight loss can be achieved with physical exercise, but that needs to exceed 225 min per week. Ross et al. demonstrated an 8% weight loss in obese men after 12 weeks of aerobic training. In the study, the men participated in daily exercise sessions of 700 kcals [45]. Similarly, the Midwest Exercise Trial showed a 5.3% weight loss after 16 weeks of aerobic exercise at approximately 2000 kcals per week [46].

Physical activity combined with diet

Studies have shown that diet modifications have a greater impact on body weight than exercise, but the combination of diet plus exercise was shown to have the greatest impact on weight loss [47]. An exercise program consistent with public health recommendations without dietary modifications leads to an average weight loss of approximately 2 kg. Although the data show that reductions in energy intake have a more significant impact on body weight than exercise, the combination of diet and exercise has the most significant impact on weight loss in short-term studies. A study in males reported an 11.4% reduction in weight after 12 weeks of diet and exercise. This can be compared to 8.4% and 0.3% in diet alone or exercise alone, respectively. For women, the weight loss was 7.5% with diet and exercise, 5.5% with diet alone, and 0.6% with exercise [48]. Other studies have shown that mean weight loss on combined diet and exercise interventions at 6 months compared to the diet-only controls were 7.8 kg, and diet only controls were 3.7 kg [49]. A metaanalysis by Miller et al. determined that the rate of weight loss was similar after caloric restriction (1.0 kg per week) and caloric restriction alone (0.98 kg per week). Weight loss by exercise alone was 0.2 kg per week [50].

Long-term weight loss and prevention of weight regain

Physical activity is essential for both weight loss and the prevention of weight gain following weight loss, but unfortunately, weight regain is extremely common [51]. The high incidence is likely because of psychological changes such as changes in appetite and hormone levels as well as the decreased resting metabolic rate. Therefore, only 20% of overweight people are able to maintain a 10% weight loss for >1 year.

Individuals who have successfully lost weight require a higher amount of physical activity to prevent weight gain. The American College of Sports Medicine emphasizes that the minimal level of physical activity to prevent weight regain is 200 min per week as compared to 150 min per week to maintain health. The National Weight Control Registry is the most extensive prospective observational study and follows individuals who have succeeded in maintaining a significant weight loss [52, 53]. The data show that high levels of physical activity are linked to successful long-term weight loss maintenance. In this study, the people who were able to maintain weight loss reported spending >60 min of moderate-intensity exercise or 35 min of high-intensity exercise per day [54–57]. Jakicic et al. reported a response between the amount of self-reported exercise per week and long-term success with weight loss at 18 months. In the study, adults who exercised >200 min per week lost more weight compared to those who exercised between 150 and 199 min per week. Similar findings were seen in women with >200 min per week after 12 months of intervention [58, 59].

References

[1] Jequier E. Pathways to obesity. Int J Obes Relat Metab Disord 2002;26(Suppl 2):S12–7.

[2] Ortega FB, Lavie CJ, Blair SN. Obesity and cardiovascular disease. Circ Res 2016;118(11):1752–70.

[3] Flatt JP. Importance of nutrient balance in body weight regulation. Diabetes Metab Rev 1988;4 (6):571–81.
[4] Ravussin E, et al. Reduced rate of energy expenditure as a risk factor for body-weight gain. N Engl J Med 1988;318(8):467–72.
[5] Astrup A, Raben A. Obesity: an inherited metabolic deficiency in the control of macronutrient balance? Eur J Clin Nutr 1992;46(9):611–20.
[6] Spiegelman BM, Flier JS. Obesity and the regulation of energy balance. Cell 2001;104 (4):531–43.
[7] Simpson SJ, Raubenheimer D. Obesity: the protein leverage hypothesis. Obes Rev 2005;6 (2):133–42.
[8] Manore MM, et al. Dynamic energy balance: an integrated framework for discussing diet and physical activity in obesity prevention—is it more than eating less and exercising more? Nutrients 2017;9(8).
[9] Hopkins M, Blundell JE. Energy balance, body composition, sedentariness and appetite regulation: pathways to obesity. Clin Sci (Lond) 2016;130(18):1615–28.
[10] Ross R. Reduction in obesity and related comorbid conditions after diet-induced weight loss or exercise-induced weight loss in men. Ann Intern Med 2000;133(2):92.
[11] Wen CP, et al. Minimum amount of physical activity for reduced mortality and extended life expectancy: a prospective cohort study. Lancet 2011;378(9798):1244–53.
[12] Marzetti E, et al. Physical activity and exercise as countermeasures to physical frailty and sarcopenia. Aging Clin Exp Res 2017;29(1):35–42.
[13] Hunter GR, et al. Exercise training and energy expenditure following weight loss. Med Sci Sports Exerc 2015;47(9):1950–7.
[14] Jakicic JM. Physical activity and weight loss. Nestle Nutr Inst Workshop Ser 2012;73:21–36.
[15] Fan JX, et al. Moderate to vigorous physical activity and weight outcomes: does every minute count? Am J Health Promot 2013;28(1):41–9.
[16] Strath SJ, et al. Objective physical activity accumulation in bouts and nonbouts and relation to markers of obesity in US adults. Prev Chronic Dis 2008;5(4):A131.
[17] Williamson DF, et al. Recreational physical activity and ten-year weight change in a US national cohort. Int J Obes Relat Metab Disord 1993;17(5):279–86.
[18] Petridou A, Siopi A, Mougios V. Exercise in the management of obesity. Metabolism 2019;92:163–9.
[19] Brown WJ, et al. Maintaining a healthy BMI. Am J Prev Med 2016;51(6):e165–78.
[20] Donnelly JE, et al. American College of Sports Medicine position stand. Appropriate physical activity intervention strategies for weight loss and prevention of weight regain for adults. Med Sci Sports Exerc 2009;41(2):459–71.
[21] Barnes JT, Elder CL, Pujol TJ. Overweight and obese adults: exercise intervention. Strength Cond J 2004;26(4):31.
[22] Jakicic JM, et al. American College of Sports Medicine position stand. Appropriate intervention strategies for weight loss and prevention of weight regain for adults. Med Sci Sports Exerc 2001;33(12):2145–56.
[23] Jensen MD, et al. 2013 AHA/ACC/TOS guideline for the management of overweight and obesity in adults: a report of the American College of Cardiology/American Heart Association Task Force on Practice Guidelines and The Obesity Society. J Am Coll Cardiol 2014;63(25 Pt B):2985–3023.
[24] Pollock ML, et al. ACSM position stand: the recommended quantity and quality of exercise for developing and maintaining cardiorespiratory and muscular fitness, and flexibility in healthy adults. Med Sci Sports Exerc 1998;30(6):975–91.

[25] Garber CE, et al. Quantity and quality of exercise for developing and maintaining cardiorespiratory, musculoskeletal, and neuromotor fitness in apparently healthy adults. Med Sci Sports Exerc 2011;43(7):1334–59.

[26] Sword DO. Exercise as a management strategy for the overweight and obese. Strength Cond J 2012;34(5):47–55.

[27] Sigal RJ, et al. Effects of aerobic training, resistance training, or both on percentage body fat and cardiometabolic risk markers in obese adolescents. JAMA Pediatr 2014;168(11):1006.

[28] Myers VH, et al. Exercise training and quality of life in individuals with type 2 diabetes: a randomized controlled trial. Diabetes Care 2013;36(7):1884–90.

[29] Swift DL, et al. Effect of different doses of aerobic exercise training on Total bilirubin levels. Med Sci Sports Exerc 2012;44(4):569–74.

[30] Church TS, et al. Effects of aerobic and resistance training on hemoglobin A1c levels in patients with type 2 diabetes. JAMA 2010;304(20):2253.

[31] Martin CK, et al. Exercise dose and quality of life. Arch Intern Med 2009;169(3):269.

[32] Kodama S. Effect of aerobic exercise training on serum levels of high-density lipoprotein cholesterol. Arch Intern Med 2007;167(10):999.

[33] Church TS, et al. Effects of different doses of physical activity on cardiorespiratory fitness among sedentary, overweight or obese postmenopausal women with elevated blood pressure. JAMA 2007;297(19):2081.

[34] Riebe D, et al. Long-term maintenance of exercise and healthy eating behaviors in overweight adults. Prev Med 2005;40(6):769–78.

[35] Byrne NM, et al. Weight loss strategies for obese adults: personalized weight management program vs. standard care. Obesity (Silver Spring) 2006;14(10):1777–88.

[36] Hills AP, Byrne NM. Physical activity in the management of obesity. Clin Dermatol 2004;22 (4):315–8.

[37] Church TS, et al. Exercise without weight loss does not reduce C-reactive protein: the INFLAME study. Med Sci Sports Exerc 2010;42(4):708–16.

[38] Hu FB. Sedentary lifestyle and risk of obesity and type 2 diabetes. Lipids 2003;38(2):103–8.

[39] Hu FB. Television watching and other sedentary behaviors in relation to risk of obesity and type 2 diabetes mellitus in women. JAMA 2003;289(14):1785.

[40] David P, et al. A walking intervention for postmenopausal women using mobile phones and interactive voice response. J Telemed Telecare 2011;18(1):20–5.

[41] Swift DL, et al. Exercise training and habitual physical activity. Am J Prev Med 2012;43 (6):629–35.

[42] Blough J, Loprinzi PD. Randomized controlled trial investigating the experimental effects of reduced habitual physical activity on cardiometabolic profile. Physiol Behav 2018;194:48–55.

[43] Richardson CR, et al. A meta-analysis of pedometer-based walking interventions and weight loss. Ann Fam Med 2008;6(1):69–77.

[44] Bravata DM, et al. Using pedometers to increase physical activity and improve health: a systematic review. JAMA 2007;298(19):2296–304.

[45] Ross R, et al. Reduction in obesity and related comorbid conditions after diet-induced weight loss or exercise-induced weight loss in men. A randomized, controlled trial. Ann Intern Med 2000;133(2):92–103.

[46] Donnelly JE, et al. Effects of 16 mo of verified, supervised aerobic exercise on macronutrient intake in overweight men and women: the Midwest exercise trial. Am J Clin Nutr 2003;78 (5):950–6.

[47] Johannsen NM, et al. Categorical analysis of the impact of aerobic and resistance exercise training, alone and in combination, on cardiorespiratory fitness levels in patients with type 2 diabetes: results from the HART-D study. Diabetes Care 2013;36(10):3305–12.

[48] Hagan RD, et al. The effects of aerobic conditioning and/or caloric restriction in overweight men and women. Med Sci Sports Exerc 1986;18(1):87–94.

[49] Wing RR. Physical activity in the treatment of the adulthood overweight and obesity: current evidence and research issues. Med Sci Sports Exerc 1999;31(11 Suppl):S547–52.

[50] Miller WC, Koceja DM, Hamilton EJ. A meta-analysis of the past 25 years of weight loss research using diet, exercise or diet plus exercise intervention. Int J Obes Relat Metab Disord 1997;21(10):941–7.

[51] Wing RR, Phelan S. Long-term weight loss maintenance. Am J Clin Nutr 2005;82 (1):222S–225S.

[52] Catenacci VA, et al. Physical activity patterns in the National Weight Control Registry. Obesity 2008;16(1):153–61.

[53] Catenacci VA, et al. Physical activity patterns using accelerometry in the National Weight Control Registry. Obesity 2010;19(6):1163–70.

[54] Dombrowski SU, et al. Long term maintenance of weight loss with non-surgical interventions in obese adults: systematic review and meta-analyses of randomised controlled trials. BMJ 2014;348:g2646.

[55] MacLean PS, et al. NIH working group report: innovative research to improve maintenance of weight loss. Obesity 2014;23(1):7–15.

[56] Anastasiou CA, Karfopoulou E, Yannakoulia M. Weight regaining: from statistics and behaviors to physiology and metabolism. Metabolism 2015;64(11):1395–407.

[57] Soleymani T, Daniel S, Garvey WT. Weight maintenance: challenges, tools and strategies for primary care physicians. Obes Rev 2015;17(1):81–93.

[58] Jakicic JM, et al. Effect of exercise duration and intensity on weight loss in overweight, sedentary women. JAMA 2003;290(10):1323.

[59] Jakicic JM, et al. Effects of intermittent exercise and use of home exercise equipment on adherence, weight loss, and fitness in overweight women. JAMA 1999;282(16):1554.

Chapter 10

Environmental factors related to the obesity epidemic

Lindsey G. Kahan, B.S. and Raman Mehrzad, M.D., M.H.L., M.B.A.
Department of Plastic and Reconstructive Surgery, Rhode Island Hospital, The Warren Alpert Medical School of Brown University, Providence, RI, United States

Introduction

Obesity is a multifactorial disease with personal, environmental, genetic, and social influences. While at its core obesity results from an excess of energy intake compared to output, the complex relationship between variables leading to both individual and population-level obesity should be better understood through an environmental lens. The way one interacts with the environment is critical to development, and understanding which factors are within one's control can help guide personal and policy initiatives. Several neighborhood-level factors have been shown to be associated with obesity, such as food availability and safety. Environmental factors within the home have also been shown to influence dietary choices, physical activity, and obesity rates. In this chapter, we will depict the environmental factors related to the obesity epidemic.

Social determinants of health

Personal behavioral patterns have the greatest contribution to premature death in the United States, accounting for about 40% (Fig. 1) [1]. The greatest behavioral factors contributing to premature death are obesity, inactivity, and smoking (Fig. 2) [1]. To develop a comprehensive understanding of the epidemiology of obesity, it is important to consider the social circumstances (15%) and environmental exposures (5%) that are related to obesity, given that these contribute to a combined 20% of premature deaths (Fig. 1).

Social circumstances refer to the environmental product of one's socioeconomic status (SES), which is comprised of income, total wealth, education, employment, and residential neighborhood. These social circumstances affect individuals, neighborhoods, and regions. Environmental exposures include

Obesity. https://doi.org/10.1016/B978-0-12-818839-2.00010-7

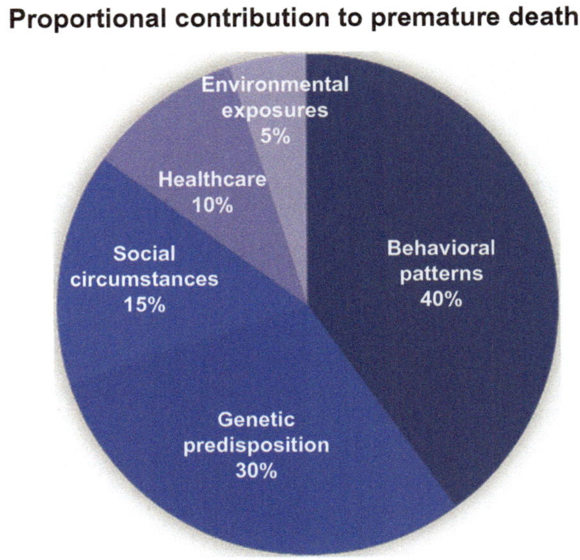

FIG. 1 The proportion of premature deaths attributable to various determinants of health. *(Adapted from Schroeder SA. We can do better—improving the health of the American people. N Engl J Med 2007 Sep;357(12):1221–1228. https://doi.org/10.1056/NEJMsa073350.)*

toxic substances such as lead paint and pollution as well as a lack of safe spaces for physical activity.

Tobacco versus obesity: A historical comparison

Through the release of scientific evidence and sweeping policy initiatives, smoking among Americans has drastically declined from 57% in 1955 to 23% in 2005, and more recently reported as 13.7% in 2018 [1, 2]. Tobacco use is a behavioral pattern that is rooted in social influences. It can be argued that the obesity epidemic is the next "big tobacco" of developed nations, and tobacco use should be analyzed as a model for tackling the obesity epidemic [1]. Smoking and obesity have many overlaps, including high prevalence, a risk factor for chronic preventable diseases, heavy use of marketing campaigns, more common in low SES areas, and difficulty in treating [1]. While obvious differences exist such as the biological need to eat, the inappropriate application of BMI to individuals compared to its intended use as a population-level tool, and the binary nature of smokers versus nonsmokers, population-wide policy changes should be scrutinized to combat the obesity epidemic [1].

Socioeconomic status

SES has been widely studied in its relationship to obesity. In developing countries, a direct relationship between SES and obesity has been shown, with a

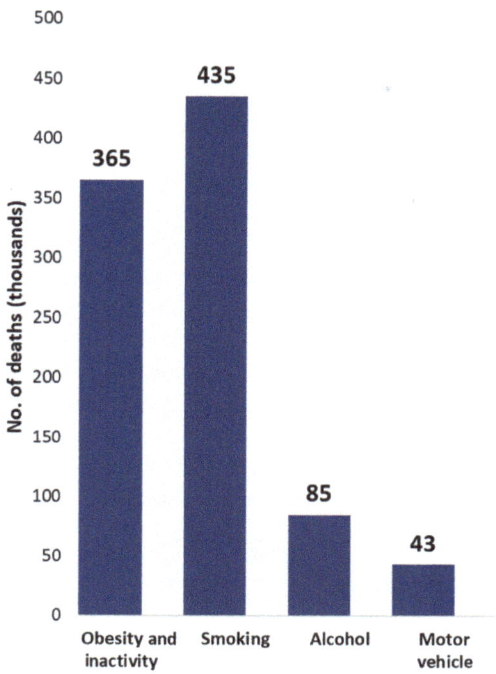

FIG. 2 The contribution of behavioral health patterns to the number of deaths in the United States, 2000. *(Adapted from Schroeder SA. We can do better—improving the health of the American people. N Engl J Med 2007 Sep;357(12):1221–1228. https://doi.org/10.1056/NEJMsa073350.)*

higher SES having a higher likelihood of having obesity [3]. Interestingly, different groups have shown different associations between BMI and obesity. For example, in a study comparing black, brown, and white Brazilian adults, it was found that men and black women had higher odds of obesity with increasing SES, yet brown and white women in the study had decreased odds of obesity with increasing SES [4]. At the lowest SES level, black women had 30% decreased odds of obesity compared to white women. At the highest SES level, black women had a three-fold increase of obesity compared to white women [4]. It was suggested that the racial disparities could be explained by a culmination of physiological, psychological, cultural, and environmental effects. Some of these potential factors include stress due to racial discrimination causing negative mental health outcomes and physiologic disturbances on the hypothalamic–pituitary–adrenal axis, or overeating secondary due to psychological distress [4].

In developed countries, an inverse relationship has been shown between BMI and obesity, more so with women than for men and children [3, 5, 6]. In a 34-article literature review of studies on SES and obesity, there were relatively consistent inverse associations between occupational status and weight gain. When income level was used as a proxy for SES, however, inconsistent findings were reported with fewer studies. In a prospective analysis of children, it was found that after controlling for ethnicity, children from lower SES families had a greater likelihood of being overweight than children of higher SES families [7].

Structural racism has led to racial inequalities in SES [8, 9], given that SES is measured through educational attainment, household income, occupation, and wealth. Structural racism, which encompasses policies and practices that white Americans have over other ethnic and racial minority groups [10], has influenced residential environments and health through disparities in home loans and housing assistance programs only historically available to whites [11–13]. These practices, of which housing disparity is a single example, have been widely shown to be associated with fewer health-promoting resources, and account for the racial differences in SES [11–15]. It is therefore important to consider structural racism in the later discussed concepts of racial/ethnic disparities in environments and their relationship to obesity.

The built environment

The environment in which one lives contributes to daily routines, community engagement, and lifestyle choices [16]. The "built environment" includes urban design, land use, transportation systems, and patterns of activity within these constructs [17]. Factors influencing the built environment can range from the density of development in an area to the aesthetic qualities of buildings and landscaping as well as the availability of public amenities (Table 1) [17].

Residents of high-walkable neighborhoods get 70 more minutes of physical activity each week and are 2.4 times more likely to meet physical activity recommendations than residents of low-walkable neighborhoods [18, 19]. Walkability has also been associated with lower BMI or reduced risk of overweight [19–21], although there are conflicting findings in the literature [22], suggesting that further work needs to be done to fully elucidate the relationship between walkability and BMI. Specifically, the county sprawl index has been shown to have significant associations with not only minutes walked, but also obesity, BMI, and hypertension [21]. Those living in an area with a greater sprawl index were less likely to walk for leisure than those in compact counties [21].

Factors in the built environment such as time spent in a car have also shown positive associations with obesity, with each additional hour in a car translating to increased odds of obesity by 6% [23]. Land use distribution was also associated with obesity. A mix of land uses within one place, specifically including residential, commercial, office, and institutional uses, was associated with a 12.2% reduction in obesity odds for each quartile increase in land use mix [23]. It has been shown that the built environment of a place influences travel

TABLE 1 The built environment consists of six qualitative and quantitative dimensions, creating a unique environment that affects individuals and communities in a region-specific manner.

Dimension	Examples
Density and intensity	Persons per acre
	Jobs per square mile
Land use mix	Distance from house to nearest store, office, or park
	Proximity measures between land area for different uses
Street connectivity	Intersections per square mile
	Average block length
Street scale	Ratio of building heights to street width
Aesthetic qualities	Often qualitative, such as building design and landscaping
	Graffiti per square mile
	Benches and lighting per square mile
Regional structure	Distribution and concentration of activities across the region
	Transportation access across the region

Adapted from Handy SL, Boarnet MG, Ewing R, Killingsworth RE. How the built environment affects physical activity. Am J Prev Med 2002 Aug;23(2):64–73. https://doi.org/10.1016/S0749-3797(02)00475-0.

and activity patterns. It has also been suggested that to increase physical activity and health, the built environment should be designed to promote walking and bicycling as methods of transportation, rather than just as exercise [17].

In recent years, the study of the built environment has been scrutinized through systematic reviews to find a potential link between environment and obesity. While there is a plethora of evidence showing associations between environmental factors and obesity, the case per the current literature for a causal relationship is less striking. The literature mainly consists of cross-sectional data rather than analyses of changes over time, which doesn't enable a comprehensive analysis of the effects of built environmental factors on changes in weight [24]. In one systematic review of the epidemiologic evidence, it was found that they could identify a concise causal role for the built environment on obesity, with the possible exception of the "county sprawl index" and the "land use mix" [25]. This limited relationship was attributed to a heterogenous body of literature, including disagreements among authors on measurements and the modeling of the built environment.

The toxic environment

The "toxic environment" represents a shift in the built environment, including social and economic changes, over the past several decades in the United States [26, 27]. The term was introduced to acknowledge and study the impact of introducing increased portion sizes, the increased prevalence and decreased cost of fast food, and a reduction in physical activity. While associations have been established, the causal nature of specific environmental exposures has yet to be fully elucidated [28]. Through the framework of one's environment, it is possible to study the individual components that lead to toxicity, such as food availability, neighborhood characteristics, and disparities among geographic locations.

Food deserts

A food desert is defined as a residential area with limited access to affordable healthy food [29]. Food deserts have been associated with obesity in America [30] and food accessibility is known to vary by a community's racial, ethnic, and socioeconomic status. The built environment is thought to explain some of the disparities in nutrition and health [16, 31] through fewer supermarkets in lower-income and minority neighborhoods [32]. It has been reported that the lowest income neighborhoods have nearly 30% fewer supermarkets than high-income neighborhoods [32a]. Even after controlling for income, disparities among race were found as well–the availability of chain supermarkets in predominantly black neighborhoods was found to be 52% of the availability of predominantly white neighborhoods [32b].

This connection is bolstered by the findings that access to supermarkets is associated with a greater intake of fruits and vegetables among participants in the US food stamp program [33] and a higher pregnancy diet quality index rating [34]. Moreover, in the most impoverished neighborhoods in Detroit, neighborhoods with a higher proportion of African Americans were on average 1.1 miles further from a supermarket than neighborhoods with a higher proportion of white residents [35]. Other studies have shown low-income neighborhoods to have half as many supermarkets as wealthier neighborhoods, fewer specialty and natural food stores, and more liquor stores [36]. Rural environments have been associated with fewer healthy and affordable food options. It has been shown that convenience stores, carrying a lesser proportion of healthful foods, significantly outnumber supermarkets and grocery stores in rural areas [37]. Not only are there fewer supermarkets in low-income areas, but healthier foods are significantly more expensive to low-income consumers as well (Fig. 3) [38].

Several studies have analyzed the relationship between food deserts and obesity. It has been shown that from a neighborhood level, food deserts are positively associated with obesity status after controlling for home food environmental factors [39]. However, it is important to consider the complexity of

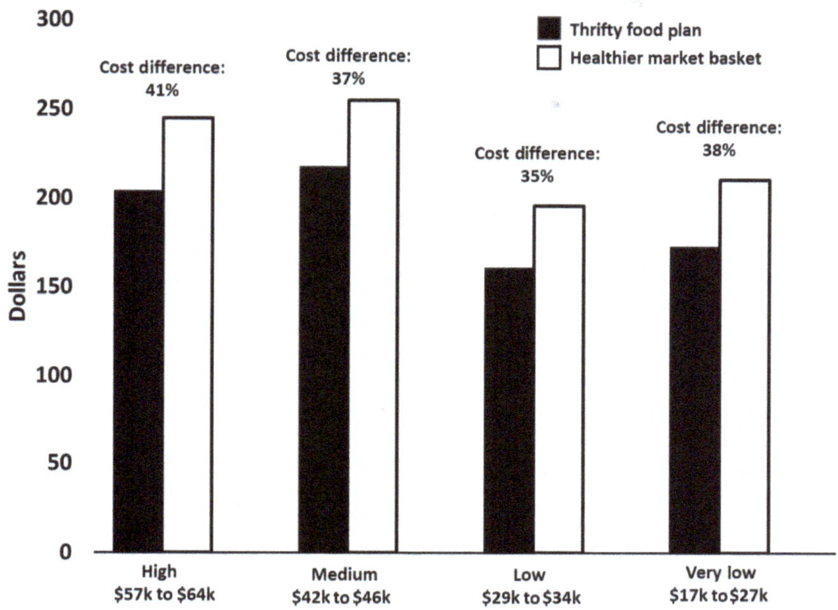

FIG. 3 Cost of the thrifty food plan versus the healthier market basket food plan in Los Angeles by neighborhood median income. The thrifty food plan consisted of foods including enriched bread, canned fruit in heavy syrup, and whole-fat dairy. The healthier market basket consisted of whole wheat bread, fruit in lite syrup, and low-fat dairy products. *(Adapted from data presented in Jetter KM, Cassady DL. The availability and cost of healthier food alternatives. Am J Prev Med 2006 Jan;30(1):38–44. https://doi.org/10.1016/j.amepre.2005.08.039.)*

this relationship from both a personal- and a population-level view while understanding the multifactorial and heterogenous nature of obesity.

While it has been established that food availability varies among regions, there remains a gap in the literature in understanding the complex and potentially causative relationship between food deserts and obesity. Data are limited by a predominance of cross-sectional studies, a lack of information about the decision-making process in purchasing patterns, and a reliance on commercial business listings, among others [40]. Future analyses should develop the relationships between factors involved with both food buying and eating choices, and use more dynamic approaches to understanding the use of other food venues such as restaurants, corner stores, and gas stations [41].

In the comparison between two food deserts through survey administration, one of which received a supermarket in the time frame between the surveys, it was found that there was no differential improvement in fruit and vegetable intake, whole grain consumption, or BMI in the supermarket group [42]. There was a reported improved perception of healthy food access in the supermarket group [42], but this study highlights the importance of considering the multifactorial nature of food choices and their affect on obesity.

The connection between food swamps, or areas with a high density of fast food and junk food [43], and obesity has mixed data in the literature. Several studies have reported no link or a modest link between fast food restaurant density and obesity [44, 45]. However, a 2017 study analyzing the relationship between food swamps, food deserts, and obesity found a significant link [46]. Food swamps were shown to not only be a separate independent phenomenon from food deserts, but were determined to potentially play a larger role than food deserts in obesity rates [46]. At the county level, food swamps were a stronger predictor of obesity than food deserts, indicating the importance of studying both the positive and negative presence of foods [46].

Urban rural divide

In the United States, the prevalence of obesity varies by region, with the South and the Midwest reporting the highest rates [47]. In developed countries, residents of rural areas are more likely to have obesity (Fig. 4) [48]. Rural residents partially attribute this to a lack of physical activity in their built environment, reporting barriers such as long travel distances to exercise facilities and unsafe roads [49]. Several factors unique to rural populations have been associated with obesity, including distance to the nearest recreational facility, an unpleasant community for physical activity, and feeling unsafe [50]. It has also been shown that residents of larger cities take more daily steps than those in smaller cities [51], potentially reflecting an overall disparity in physical activity between environments.

It has been reported that increases in global BMI have paralleled the increasing population in cities, leading to the notion that urbanization is a main driver of the global rise in obesity [52–54]. However, it was found that globally, 55% of BMI increases can be attributed to rural areas, and this percentage increases to 60–90% in the rural regions of low- and middle-income countries, including regions of sub-Saharan Africa; east, south, and southeast Asia; and Oceania [55]. In contrast, urbanization contributed significantly less to the rise of BMI. Low- and middle-income countries were shown to have the greatest rate of BMI increase in rural areas, leading to a convergence of the BMIs of those in urban and rural environments (Fig. 4) [55]. In emerging economies in South Asia, rural communities were found to be responsible for 86% of the BMI rise in men, whereas urban communities were responsible for only 8% (Fig. 5). This is in contrast with high-income Asia Pacific regions, which attributed 72% of the BMI rise in men to urban environments. The process of urbanization throughout both low- and high-income areas did not contribute as much to BMI rise in men as rural or urban areas separately (Fig. 5) [55].

Neighborhood characteristics

Community resources are associated with self-identified racial, ethnic, and socioeconomic factors [56]. Across the United States, physical activity-related

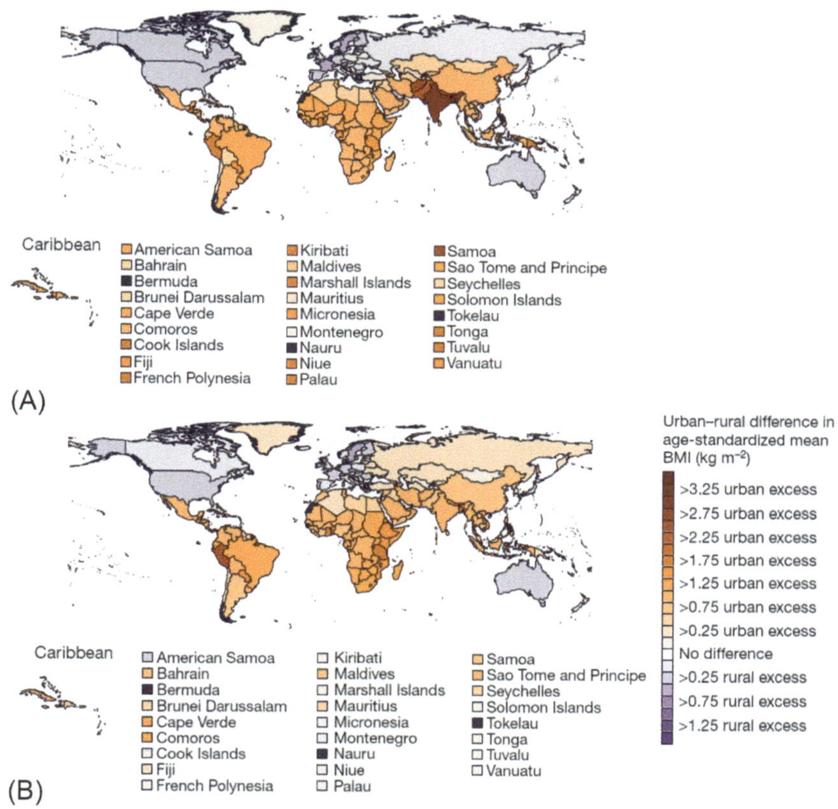

FIG. 4 The difference between rural and urban age-standardized mean BMI in men. (A) Difference in age-standardized mean BMI in 1985 compared to (B) difference in age-standardized mean BMI in 2017. *(Reproduced with permission from NCD Risk Factor Collaboration (NCD-RisC). Rising rural body-mass index is the main driver of the global obesity epidemic in adults. Nature 2019 May;569(7755):260–264. https://doi.org/10.1038/s41586-019-1171-x.)*

facilities were found to be less likely to be present in lower-income neighborhoods [57]. This disparity extends to influencing self-identified racial/ethnic groups, with physical activity-related facilities being less likely to be present in communities with higher proportions of African American, Hispanic, and other minority residents [57]. Socioeconomically, compared to a community with a median income level of \$25,000, a community with a median income level of \$75,000 was found to have a higher likelihood of physical fitness facilities, membership sports clubs, dance facilities, and public golf courses by 17%, 38%, 30%, and 54%, respectively [57]. Low- and medium-socioeconomic status neighborhoods also have significantly fewer free-for-use resources than high-socioeconomic status neighborhoods [58].

Environmental factors have been associated with the proportion of residents who are overweight in Nigeria when controlled for socioeconomic status [59].

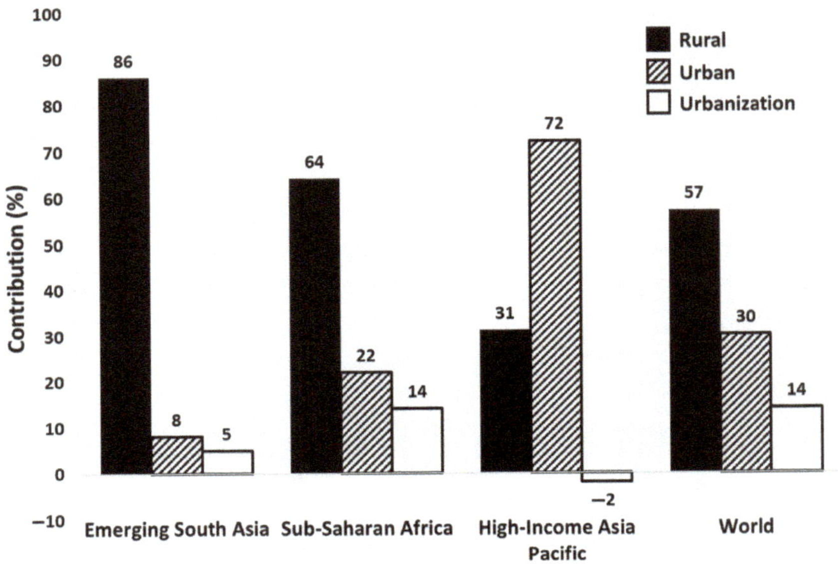

FIG. 5 Contributors to the rise in mean BMI in men from 1985 to 2017 in selected populations. *(Adapted from data presented in NCD Risk Factor Collaboration (NCD-RisC). Rising rural body-mass index is the main driver of the global obesity epidemic in adults. Nature 2019 May;569 (7755):260–264. https://doi.org/10.1038/s41586-019-1171-x.)*

Specifically, the distance to commercial facilities, poor neighborhood aesthetics, perceived garbage in the neighborhood, and unsafe feelings were all associated with overweight [59]. In Korea, there has been an association between a higher satisfaction with safety and public transportation, accessibility to sports facilities, and lower obesity risk [60].

In a study among adults in Missouri, similar environmental factors were associated with overweight, including unsafe and unpleasant community perceptions and the lack of outdoor exercise facilities [61]. Other studies have corroborated these findings, reporting significant associations between obesity and the perception of an unpleasant community, lack of interesting sites, poor sidewalk quality, and the presence of garbage [62]. These studies show the ubiquitous and global nature of neighborhood qualities and their associations to obesity.

Starting young: Obesity through pediatrics

Home life factors

Personal behavioral patterns are influenced by social and environmental factors. This is particularly relevant for the analysis of childhood obesity, given that children have had less time and exposure to factors outside their home environments to influence their food choices or weight. Moreover, childhood obesity is a critical disease to understand, given that children with obesity are more likely to have obesity as adults, with about half of school-aged children with obesity being afflicted by adult obesity [63].

The analysis of groups of children can isolate patterns of behavior that may contribute to obesity. For example, when stratified by self-identified race/ethnicity, it was found that Latino children exhibit a higher prevalence of overweight (47%) and obesity (31%) compared to white children (35% and 21%, respectively) [64].

Parental influences

Parenting style has frequently been studied in terms of its influence on weight-related behaviors and health [65–68]. Classically described parenting styles include authoritative, authoritarian, permissive, and neglectful [69, 70]. Parenting styles are based on the degree of responsiveness and the degree of demandingness of the parent, with authoritative parenting displaying high degrees of both; the other three parenting styles display some combination of low and high degrees of responsiveness and demandingness. It has been suggested that authoritative parenting provides the required structure and support for positive behaviors, including the regulation of eating [65, 71]. Several cross-sectional studies have identified the authoritative parenting style as having a higher association with lower youth BMI, more frequent physical activity, and healthy dietary intake [72–75]. One longitudinal study in an ethnically and socioeconomi cally diverse population found that material authoritative parenting may have a protective role in children's BMI over time [65].

Other aspects of parental influences have also been studied to understand relationships between the home environment and weight. The role of family functioning, or the structural and organizational aspects and interpersonal relationships within the home, influences child development. Higher family functioning, as assessed by the Family Assessment Device [76, 77], has shown significant association with more frequent family meals in both adolescent girls and boys after adjusting for age, SES, and race/ethnicity [67]. Modest association was shown between higher family functioning and greater intake of fruits and vegetables, lower BMI, and lower percent overweight in girls [67].

The study of family meals has been particularly revealing of child behavior and health. Cross-sectional results have shown that the authoritative parenting style has been associated with the frequency of family meals [66]. Longitudinal results showed that authoritative parenting predicted a higher frequency of family meals 5 years later in opposite sex parent/adolescent dyads [66]. Family meal frequency has been associated with a lower risk of underintake of vegetables and fruits, and those with a higher frequency of family meals were less likely to skip breakfast [78]. Moreover, it has been shown that family meals during adolescence, at any frequency, were significantly associated with reduced overweight and obesity as young adults [68].

Permissive and indulgent parenting styles, characterized by low demands yet ample warmth and sensitivity, have been associated with the highest child BMIs [79–81]. Self-identified Latino populations have reported higher rates of permissive and indulgent parenting styles [82], potentially contributing to the increased prevalence of overweight and obesity in Latino children. Other factors studied within the Latino population include a high reported prevalence of pressure-to-eat feeding practice, leading to increased food consumption [83, 84].

Screen time

The increase in screen time for young children demonstrates a generational divide in child-rearing practices due to the increased availability of technology in the home in the form of tablets, phones, and computers. Preschoolers are an important group of children to study due to the known relationship between early childhood education and future cognitive growth, higher health outcomes, increased likelihood of high school graduation, and higher income [85–87]. One study reported that in 2011, preschoolers spent an average of 4.1 h per day using a screen [88], and another group found this average to be 5.1 ± 3.6h a day in 2019 [89]. Excessive screen time has been associated with elevated BMI in preschoolers [90–92]. In 2002, 40% of preschoolers in a US-based study reported a TV in their bedroom, and these children were more likely to be overweight [92].

Moreover, screen time has been found to vary based on race/ethnicity within the preschool population, with black and Hispanic children reporting higher average screen times than white children [92]. This suggests a potential environmental disadvantage for nonwhite children in maintaining a healthy BMI. In the only screen time and child weight status study in low- and middle-income countries, it was found that higher screen time on weekends was associated with higher BMI in a Brazilian population after controlling for household income, parental occupation, and parental BMI [93].

School-aged children and adolescents are other vulnerable age groups when analyzing the relationship between screen time and weight. It has been shown that dietary behaviors and screen time often cooccur in a clustered synergistic manner [94–96]. Not only are children exposed to unhealthy food advertisements that can influence food consumption and BMI [97], but watching TV can cause distraction and a lack of awareness of food consumption, leading to overconsumption [98].

Racial/ethnic divides, particularly among first-generation immigrant Spanish-speaking families, have been studied within the context of television watching. Parents were reported to encourage their children to watch TV for English speech and language improvement [82]. While potentially holding educational value, the encouragement of TV watching potentially increases screen time, decreases physical activity, and increases time exposed to unhealthy food advertisements. While fewer food advertisements were shown on Spanish-language channels in the United States, when analyzed for nutritional content, the food products advertised on Spanish-language channels were substantially more unhealthy than those on English-language channels [99]. The rates of TVs in bedrooms also vary with race/ethnicity in children and adolescents, with 74% of Latino children and 70% of black children reporting having a TV in their bedroom, compared to 22% of white children having a TV where they slept [100].

Preschool and health outcomes

Early childhood development interventions have an increasing amount of evidence in proving short- and long-term benefits, including improved cognitive development and school success [86]. Children who participated in Head Start programs, which include a preschool with nutritional education services and healthy food options, had a 24.9% reduction in the probability of being overweight [101]. Compared to self-identified black children who did not attend Head Start, those who attended had an overweight reduction of 33.4% between the ages of 5 and 19 [101]. Other studies have corroborated these results at older grades, and have reported that Head Start participation in the third and fifth grades has had significant positive effects on reducing the risk of overweight/obesity [102]. It has been postulated that the nutrition, health care, and parental involvement in Head Start programs contribute to the decreased risk of obesity.

Physical activity

The US Department of Health and Human Services recommends 60min or more of moderate to vigorous daily physical activity, including aerobic, muscle-strengthening, and bone-strengthening exercises [103]. Increased physical activity has consistently been shown to reduce all-cause mortality, and inactivity and underactivity compared to recommended guidelines have been shown to contribute to years of life lost. This loss increases as weight increases, with a loss of 7.2years of life for inactive adults with obesity class II (Fig. 6) [104]. Moreover, only 23% of children ages 6 to 17 meet the recommended guidelines, with 9.5% participating in zero days per week of 60min of physical activity [105]. Physical activity also varies by ethnicity and sex, with minority adolescents and females reporting the lowest levels of vigorous activity [106].

A lack of physical activity has frequently been associated with childhood obesity, and engagement in sports and exercise programs is associated with a decreased chance of childhood overweight [107–109]. One longitudinal study of the association between change in BMI and physical activity in children over time found that an increase in physical activity was associated with decreasing relative BMI in girls and overweight boys [110].

Several factors influence the level of physical activity of different groups, such as availability, neighborhood safety, leisure time, and expense [111]. Lower levels of neighborhood safety have been associated with decreased

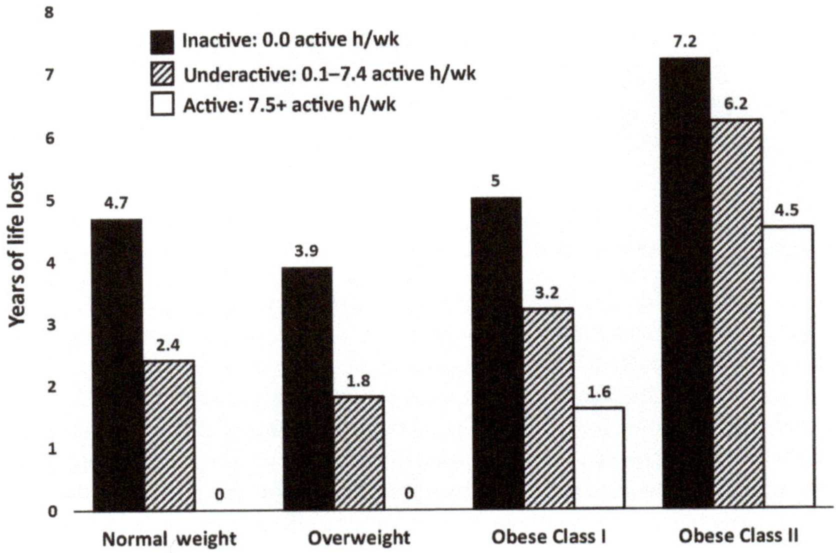

FIG. 6 Years of life lost after age 40 in relation to activity level as varied by BMI. US guidelines recommend 7.5 or greater metabolic equivalent hours per week of physical activity. Normal weight is a BMI of 18.5–24.9 kg/m^2, overweight is a BMI of 25.0–29.9 kg/m^2, obese class I is a BMI of 30.0–34.9 kg/m^2, and obese class II is a BMI of 35.0 kg/m^2 or greater. *(Adapted from Moore SC, et al. Leisure time physical activity of moderate to vigorous intensity and mortality: a large pooled cohort analysis. PLoS Med 2012 Nov;9(11). https://doi.org/10.1371/journal.pmed.1001335.)*

physical activity and higher rates of obesity [112]. This has been especially true in Latino population due to the aforementioned challenges in exposing their children to physical activity. It has been found that there is a strong correlation between inactivity and time spent watching TV, and Latino children in lower-income communities and unsafe neighborhoods were more likely to be physically inactive and overweight [82, 111].

Sleep duration

Children's sleep patterns have been studied in relationship to obesity risk. Studies have reported that sleeping less than the recommended amount during early childhood is an independent and strong risk factor for both childhood and adult obesity [113, 114]. Even 1 h less of sleep per night in preadolescent Canadian children was associated with an increased odds ratio of being overweight or obese [115]. In Latino children under the age of 13, it was shown that Latino children sleep less than 9 h a day, significantly less than the recommendation of 10–11 h a day [82, 116]. It was also found that children with obesity slept less than children within a normal weight [116]. In a sample of Portuguese children ages 7–9, it was found that the prevalence of overweight/obesity decreased with long sleep duration [117]. Moreover, lower parental education level, increased TV watching, and decreased physical activity were all associated with less sleep [117]. These latter associations highlight the importance of environmental factors when considering the pathogenesis of obesity.

Immigration and obesity

It is known that immigrants to the United States are healthier than the native population, and with time and generations, their health outcomes converge to that of native-born Americans [118]. This phenomenon is termed the *healthy immigrant effect*. Average immigrant BMIs are 2% and 5% points lower than native-born females and males, respectively [119]. Within 10 years of arrival, female immigrant BMIs converge with those of native-born females [119]. In addition to time, the assimilation of environmental factors was associated with BMI. For example, a female immigrant's English language skills were significantly correlated with an increase in BMI [118], and this corroborates other literature that showed language assimilation as a predictor of obesity [120].

Other studies have also shown the healthy immigrant effect to occur in Canada, where after 20–30 years, immigrant weight meets or exceeds native-born weight [121]. Protective immigration factors were also identified, such as less weight gain if an immigrant resides within a significant ethnic social network where the ethnic community is less likely to be overweight [121].

Summary

While the pathogenesis of obesity is multifactorial, the data clearly indicate that there is a relationship between environmental factors and obesity. Several associations have been represented throughout the literature between the built environment and rates of obesity. Obesity has been shown to vary with both macro- and microenvironmental factors, including food availability, neighborhood safety, and parental influence. While causality has been harder to prove in the literature, several studies have indicated that early interventions, increased access to healthy food and physical activity, and increased parental guidance can reduce rates of obesity.

References

[1] Schroeder SA. We can do better—improving the health of the American people. N Engl J Med 2007 Sep;357(12):1221–8. https://doi.org/10.1056/NEJMsa073350.

[2] Creamer MR, et al. Tobacco product use and cessation indicators among adults—United States, 2018. Morb Mortal Wkly Rep 2019 Nov;68(45):1013–9. https://doi.org/10.15585/mmwr.mm6845a2.

[3] Sobal J, Stunkard AJ. Socioeconomic status and obesity: a review of the literature. Psychol Bull 1989;105(2):260–75. https://doi.org/10.1037/0033-2909.105.2.260.

[4] Araujo MC, Baltar VT, Yokoo EM, Sichieri R. The association between obesity and race among Brazilian adults is dependent on sex and socio-economic status. Public Health Nutr 2018 Aug;21(11):2096–102. https://doi.org/10.1017/S1368980018000307.

[5] Ball K, Crawford D. Socioeconomic status and weight change in adults: a review. Soc Sci Med 2005 May;60(9):1987–2010. https://doi.org/10.1016/j.socscimed.2004.08.056.

[6] Jeffery RW, Forster JL, Folsom AR, Luepker RV, Jacobs DR, Blackburn H. The relationship between social status and body mass index in the Minnesota Heart Health Program. Int J Obes (Lond) 1989;13(1):59–67.

[7] Goodman E. The role of socioeconomic status gradients in explaining differences in US adolescents' health. Am J Public Health 1999 Oct;89(10):1522–8. https://doi.org/10.2105/AJPH.89.10.1522.

[8] Williams DR, Priest N, Anderson NB. Understanding associations among race, socioeconomic status, and health: patterns and prospects. Health Psychol 2016 Apr;35(4):407–11. https://doi.org/10.1037/hea0000242.

[9] Phillips C. Institutional racism and ethnic inequalities: an expanded multilevel framework. J Soc Policy 2011 Jan;40(1):173–92. https://doi.org/10.1017/S0047279410000565.

[10] Bell CN, Kerr J, Young JL. Associations between obesity, obesogenic environments, and structural racism vary by county-level racial composition. Int J Environ Res Public Health 2019 Mar;16(5). https://doi.org/10.3390/ijerph16050861.

[11] Kramer MR, Hogue CR. Is segregation bad for your health? Epidemiol Rev 2009;31:178–94. https://doi.org/10.1093/epirev/mxp001.

[12] White K, Borrell LN. Racial/ethnic residential segregation: framing the context of health risk and health disparities. Health Place 2011 Mar;17(2):438–48. https://doi.org/10.1016/j.healthplace.2010.12.002.

[13] Williams DR, Collins C. Racial residential segregation: a fundamental cause of racial disparities in health. Public Health Rep (1974) 2001 Oct;116(5):404–16. https://doi.org/10.1093/phr/116.5.404.

[14] Corral I, Landrine H, Hao Y, Zhao L, Mellerson JL, Cooper DL. Residential segregation, health behavior and overweight/obesity among a national sample of African American adults. J Health Psychol 2012 Apr;17(3):371–8. https://doi.org/10.1177/1359105311417191.

[15] Bleich SN, Thorpe RJ, Sharif-Harris H, Fesahazion R, Laveist TA. Social context explains race disparities in obesity among women. J Epidemiol Community Health 2010 May;64(5):465–9. https://doi.org/10.1136/jech.2009.096297.

[16] Sallis JF, Glanz K. The role of built environments in physical activity, eating, and obesity in childhood. Future Child 2006;16(1):89–108. https://doi.org/10.1353/foc.2006.0009.

[17] Handy SL, Boarnet MG, Ewing R, Killingsworth RE. How the built environment affects physical activity. Am J Prev Med 2002 Aug;23(2):64–73. https://doi.org/10.1016/S0749-3797(02)00475-0.

[18] Frank LD, Schmid TL, Sallis JF, Chapman J, Saelens BE. Linking objectively measured physical activity with objectively measured urban form. Am J Prev Med 2005 Feb;28(2):117–25. https://doi.org/10.1016/j.amepre.2004.11.001.

[19] Saelens BE, Sallis JF, Black JB, Chen D. Neighborhood-based differences in physical activity: an environment scale evaluation. Am J Public Health 2003 Sep;93(9):1552–8. https://doi.org/10.2105/AJPH.93.9.1552.

[20] Giles-Corti B, Macintyre S, Clarkson JP, Pikora T, Donovan RJ. Environmental and lifestyle factors associated with overweight and obesity in Perth, Australia. Am J Health Promot 2003 Sep;18(1):93–102. https://doi.org/10.4278/0890-1171-18.1.93.

[21] Ewing R, Schmid T, Killingsworth R, Zlot A, Raudenbush S. Relationship between urban sprawl and physical activity, obesity, and morbidity. Am J Health Promot 2003 Sep;18 (1):47–57. https://doi.org/10.4278/0890-1171-18.1.47.

[22] Norman GJ, Nutter SK, Ryan S, Sallis JF, Calfas KJ, Patrick K. Community design and access to recreational facilities as correlates of adolescent physical activity and body-mass index. J Phys Act Health 2006 Feb;3(s1):S118–28. https://doi.org/10.1123/jpah.3.s1.s118.

[23] Frank LD, Andresen MA, Schmid TL. Obesity relationships with community design, physical activity, and time spent in cars. Am J Prev Med 2004 Aug;27(2):87–96. https://doi.org/10.1016/j.amepre.2004.04.011.

[24] Sturm R, An R. Obesity and economic environments: obesity and economic environments. CA Cancer J Clin 2014 Sep;64(5):337–50. https://doi.org/10.3322/caac.21237.

[25] Feng J, Glass TA, Curriero FC, Stewart WF, Schwartz BS. The built environment and obesity: a systematic review of the epidemiologic evidence. Health Place 2010 Mar;16(2):175–90. https://doi.org/10.1016/j.healthplace.2009.09.008.

[26] Battle EK, Brownell KD. Confronting a rising tide of eating disorders and obesity: treatment vs. prevention and policy. Addict Behav 1996 Nov;21(6):755–65. https://doi.org/10.1016/0306-4603(96)00034-2.

[27] Faith MS, Kral TVE. Social environmental and genetic influences on obesity and obesity-promoting behaviors: fostering research integration. National Academies Press (US); 2006.

[28] Jeffery RW, Utter J. The changing environment and population obesity in the United States. Obes Res 2003 Oct;11(S10):12S–22S. https://doi.org/10.1038/oby.2003.221.

[29] Ver Ploeg M, et al. Access to affordable and nutritious food: Measuring and understanding food deserts and their consequences. Washington, DC: United States Department of Agriculture Economic Research Service; 2009.

[30] Morland K, Diez Roux AV, Wing S. Supermarkets, other food stores, and obesity. Am J Prev Med 2006 Apr;30(4):333–9. https://doi.org/10.1016/j.amepre.2005.11.003.

[31] Larson N, Story M. A review of environmental influences on food choices. Ann Behav Med 2009 Dec;38(S1):56–73. https://doi.org/10.1007/s12160-009-9120-9.

[32] Morland K, Wing S, Diez Roux A, Poole C. Neighborhood characteristics associated with the location of food stores and food service places. Am J Prev Med 2002 Jan;22(1):23–9. https://doi.org/10.1016/S0749-3797(01)00403-2.

[32a] Weinberg Z. No place to shop: the lack of supermarkets in low-income neighborhoods: analysis of a University of Connecticut study on low-income communities and households receiving public assistance in 21 metropolitan areas. Washington, DC: Public Voice for Food and Health Policy; 1995.

[32b] Powell LM, Slater S, Mirtcheva D, Bao Y, Chaloupka FJ. Food store availability and neighborhood characteristics in the United States. Prev Med 2007;44(3):189–95. https://doi.org/10.1016/j.ypmed.2006.08.008.

[33] Rose D, Richards R. Food store access and household fruit and vegetable use among participants in the US Food Stamp Program. Public Health Nutr 2004 Dec;7(8):1081–8. https://doi.org/10.1079/PHN2004648.

[34] Laraia B. Proximity of supermarkets is positively associated with diet quality index for pregnancy. Prev Med 2004 Nov;39(5):869–75. https://doi.org/10.1016/j.ypmed.2004.03.018.

[35] Zenk SN, Schulz AJ, Israel BA, James SA, Bao S, Wilson ML. Neighborhood racial composition, neighborhood poverty, and the spatial accessibility of supermarkets in metropolitan Detroit. Am J Public Health 2005 Apr;95(4):660–7. https://doi.org/10.2105/AJPH.2004.042150.

[36] Moore LV, Diez Roux AV. Associations of neighborhood characteristics with the location and type of food stores. Am J Public Health 2006 Feb;96(2):325–31. https://doi.org/10.2105/AJPH.2004.058040.

[37] Liese AD, Weis KE, Pluto D, Smith E, Lawson A. Food store types, availability, and cost of foods in a rural environment. J Am Diet Assoc 2007 Nov;107(11):1916–23. https://doi.org/10.1016/j.jada.2007.08.012.

[38] Jetter KM, Cassady DL. The availability and cost of healthier food alternatives. Am J Prev Med 2006 Jan;30(1):38–44. https://doi.org/10.1016/j.amepre.2005.08.039.

[39] Chen D, Jaenicke EC, Volpe RJ. Food environments and obesity: household diet expenditure versus food deserts. Am J Public Health 2016 May;106(5):881–8. https://doi.org/10.2105/AJPH.2016.303048.

[40] Gordon-Larsen P. Food availability/convenience and obesity. Adv Nutr 2014 Nov;5(6):809–17. https://doi.org/10.3945/an.114.007070.

[41] Walker RE, Keane CR, Burke JG. Disparities and access to healthy food in the United States: a review of food deserts literature. Health Place 2010 Sep;16(5):876–84. https://doi.org/10.1016/j.healthplace.2010.04.013.

[42] Dubowitz T, et al. Diet and perceptions change with supermarket introduction in a food desert, but not because of supermarket use. Health Affairs 2015 Nov;34(11):1858–68. https://doi.org/10.1377/hlthaff.2015.0667.

[43] Rose D, Bodor JN, Swalm C, Rice J, Farley T, Hutchinson P. Deserts in New Orleans? Illustrations of urban food access and implications for policy. Tulane University, New Orleans, LA: School of Public Health and Tropical Medicine; 2009.

[44] Maddock J. The relationship between obesity and the prevalence of fast food restaurants: state-level analysis. Am J Health Promot 2004 Nov;19(2):137–43. https://doi.org/10.4278/0890-1171-19.2.137.

[45] Simmons D, et al. Choice and availability of takeaway and restaurant food is not related to the prevalence of adult obesity in rural communities in Australia. Int J Obes (Lond) 2005 Jun;29(6):703–10. https://doi.org/10.1038/sj.ijo.0802941.

[46] Cooksey-Stowers K, Schwartz M, Brownell K. Food swamps predict obesity rates better than food deserts in the United States. Int J Environ Res Public Health 2017 Nov;14(11):1366. https://doi.org/10.3390/ijerph14111366.

[47] Gurka MJ, Filipp SL, DeBoer MD. Geographical variation in the prevalence of obesity, metabolic syndrome, and diabetes among US adults. Nutr Diabetes 2018 Dec;8(1):14. https://doi.org/10.1038/s41387-018-0024-2.

[48] Lenardson JD, Hansen AY, Hartley D. Rural and remote food environments and obesity. Curr Obes Rep 2015 Mar;4(1):46–53. https://doi.org/10.1007/s13679-014-0136-5.

[49] Seguin R, Connor L, Nelson M, LaCroix A, Eldridge G. Understanding barriers and facilitators to healthy eating and active living in rural communities. J Nutr Metab 2014;2014:1–8. https://doi.org/10.1155/2014/146502.

[50] Boehmer TK, Lovegreen SL, Haire-Joshu D, Brownson RC. What constitutes an obesogenic environment in rural communities? Am J Health Promot 2006 Jul;20(6):411–21. https://doi.org/10.4278/0890-1171-20.6.411.

[51] Ihara M, et al. A cross-sectional study of the association between city scale and daily steps in Japan: data from the National Health and Nutrition Survey Japan (NHNS-J) 2006–2010. Nihon Koshu Eisei Zasshi 2016;63(9):549–59. https://doi.org/10.11236/jph.63.9_549.

[52] World Health Organization and UN-Habitat, Global report on urban health: equitable, healthier cities for sustainable development. Geneva: World Health Organization; 2016.

[53] Wagner K-H, Brath H. A global view on the development of non communicable diseases. Prev Med 2012 May;54:S38–41. https://doi.org/10.1016/j.ypmed.2011.11.012.

[54] Popkin BM. Global nutrition dynamics: the world is shifting rapidly toward a diet linked with noncommunicable diseases. Am J Clin Nutr 2006 Aug;84(2):289–98. https://doi.org/10.1093/ajcn/84.2.289.

[55] NCD Risk Factor Collaboration (NCD-RisC). Rising rural body-mass index is the main driver of the global obesity epidemic in adults. Nature 2019 May;569(7755):260–4. https://doi.org/10.1038/s41586-019-1171-x.

[56] Powell L, Slater S, Chaloupka F. The relationship between community physical activity settings and race, ethnicity and socioeconomic status. Evidence Based Prev Med 2004;1(2).

[57] Powell LM, Slater S, Chaloupka FJ, Harper D. Availability of physical activity-related facilities and neighborhood demographic and socioeconomic characteristics: a national study. Am J Public Health 2006 Sep;96(9):1676–80. https://doi.org/10.2105/AJPH.2005.065573.

[58] Estabrooks PA, Lee RE, Gyurcsik NC. Resources for physical activity participation: does availability and accessibility differ by neighborhood socioeconomic status? Ann Behav Med 2003 Apr;25(2):100–4. https://doi.org/10.1207/S15324796ABM2502_05.

[59] Oyeyemi AL, Adegoke BO, Oyeyemi AY, Deforche B, Bourdeaudhuij I, Sallis JF. Environmental factors associated with overweight among adults in Nigeria. Int J Behav Nutr Phys Act 2012;9(1):32. https://doi.org/10.1186/1479-5868-9-32.

[60] Yoon N-H, Kwon S. The effects of community environment factors on obesity among Korean adults: a multi-level analysis. Epidemiol Health 2014 Dec;e2014036. https://doi.org/10.4178/epih/e2014036.

[61] Catlin TK, Simoes EJ, Brownson RC. Environmental and policy factors associated with overweight among adults in Missouri. Am J Health Promot 2003 Mar;17(4):249–58. https://doi.org/10.4278/0890-1171-17.4.249.

[62] Boehmer TK, Hoehner CM, Deshpande AD, Brennan Ramirez LK, Brownson RC. Perceived and observed neighborhood indicators of obesity among urban adults. Int J Obes (Lond) 2007 Jun;31(6):968–77. https://doi.org/10.1038/sj.ijo.0803531.

[63] Serdula MK, Ivery D, Coates RJ, Freedman DS, Williamson DF, Byers T. Do obese children become obese adults? A review of the literature. Prev Med 1993 Mar;22(2):167–77. https://doi.org/10.1006/pmed.1993.1014.

[64] Flores G, Tomany-Korman SC. Racial and ethnic disparities in medical and dental health, access to care, and use of services in US children. Pediatrics 2008 Jan;121(2):e286–98. https://doi.org/10.1542/peds.2007-1243.

[65] Berge JM, Wall M, Loth K, Neumark-Sztainer D. Parenting style as a predictor of adolescent weight and weight-related behaviors. J Adolesc Health 2010 Apr;46(4):331–8. https://doi.org/10.1016/j.jadohealth.2009.08.004.

[66] Berge JM, Wall M, Neumark-Sztainer D, Larson N, Story M. Parenting style and family meals: cross-sectional and 5-year longitudinal associations. J Am Diet Assoc 2010 Jul;110(7):1036–42. https://doi.org/10.1016/j.jada.2010.04.011.

[67] Berge JM, Wall M, Larson N, Loth KA, Neumark-Sztainer D. Family functioning: associations with weight status, eating behaviors, and physical activity in adolescents. J Adolesc Health 2013 Mar;52(3):351–7. https://doi.org/10.1016/j.jadohealth.2012.07.006.

[68] Berge JM, Wall M, Hsueh T-F, Fulkerson JA, Larson N, Neumark-Sztainer D. The protective role of family meals for youth obesity: 10-year longitudinal associations. J Pediatr 2015 Feb;166(2):296–301. https://doi.org/10.1016/j.jpeds.2014.08.030.

[69] Darling N, Steinberg L. Parenting style as context: an integrative model. Psychol Bull 1993;113(3):487–96. https://doi.org/10.1037/0033-2909.113.3.487.

[70] Damon W, editor. Child development today and tomorrow. 1st ed. San Francisco: Jossey-Bass Publishers; 1989.

[71] Rhee KE. Parenting styles and overweight status in first grade. Pediatrics 2006 Jun;117(6):2047–54. https://doi.org/10.1542/peds.2005-2259.

[72] Arredondo EM, Elder JP, Ayala GX, Campbell N, Baquero B, Duerksen S. Is parenting style related to children's healthy eating and physical activity in Latino families? Health Educ Res 2006 Dec;21(6):862–71. https://doi.org/10.1093/her/cyl110.

[73] Kremers SPJ, Brug J, de Vries H, Engels RCME. Parenting style and adolescent fruit consumption. Appetite 2003 Aug;41(1):43–50. https://doi.org/10.1016/s0195-6663(03)00038-2.

[74] Mellin AE, Neumark-Sztainer D, Story M, Ireland M, Resnick MD. Unhealthy behaviors and psychosocial difficulties among overweight adolescents: the potential impact of familial factors. J Adolesc Health 2002 Aug;31(2):145–53. https://doi.org/10.1016/s1054-139x(01)00396-2.

[75] Berge JM, Wall M, Bauer KW, Neumark-Sztainer D. Parenting characteristics in the home environment and adolescent overweight: a latent class analysis. Obesity 2010 Apr;18(4):818–25. https://doi.org/10.1038/oby.2009.324.

[76] Miller IW, Epstein NB, Bishop DS, Keitner GI. The McMaster Family Assessment Device: reliability and validity. J Marital Fam Ther 1985 Oct;11(4):345–56. https://doi.org/10.1111/j.1752-0606.1985.tb00028.x.

[77] Epstein NB, Baldwin LM, Bishop DS. The McMaster Family Assessment Device. J Marital Fam Ther 1983 Apr;9(2):171–80. https://doi.org/10.1111/j.1752-0606.1983.tb01497.x.

[78] Videon TM, Manning CK. Influences on adolescent eating patterns: the importance of family meals. J Adolesc Health 2003 May;32(5):365–73. https://doi.org/10.1016/S1054-139X(02)00711-5.

[79] Olvera N, Power TG. Brief report: parenting styles and obesity in Mexican American children: a longitudinal study. J Pediatr Psychol 2010 Apr;35(3):243–9. https://doi.org/10.1093/jpepsy/jsp071.

[80] Hughes SO, Shewchuk RM, Baskin ML, Nicklas TA, Qu H. Indulgent feeding style and children's weight status in preschool. J Dev Behav Pediatr 2008 Oct;29(5):403–10. https://doi.org/10.1097/DBP.0b013e318182a976.

[81] Hughes SO, Power TG, Orlet Fisher J, Mueller S, Nicklas TA. Revisiting a neglected construct: parenting styles in a child-feeding context. Appetite 2005 Feb;44(1):83–92. https://doi.org/10.1016/j.appet.2004.08.007.

[82] Ochoa A, Berge JM. Home environmental influences on childhood obesity in the Latino population: a decade review of literature. J Immigr Minor Health 2017 Apr;19(2):430–47. https://doi.org/10.1007/s10903-016-0539-3.

[83] Evans A, et al. Parental feeding practices and concerns related to child underweight, picky eating, and using food to calm differ according to ethnicity/race, acculturation, and income. Matern Child Health J 2011 Oct;15(7):899–909. https://doi.org/10.1007/s10995-009-0526-6.

[84] Martinez SM, Rhee K, Blanco E, Boutelle K. Maternal attitudes and behaviors regarding feeding practices in elementary school-aged Latino children: a pilot qualitative study on the impact of the cultural role of mothers in the US-Mexican border region of San Diego, California. J Acad Nutr Diet 2014 Feb;114(2):230–7. https://doi.org/10.1016/j.jand.2013.09.028.

[85] Ready DD. Socioeconomic disadvantage, school attendance, and early cognitive development: the differential effects of school exposure. Sociol Educ 2010;8(4):271–86.

[86] D'Onise K, Lynch JW, Sawyer MG, McDermott RA. Can preschool improve child health outcomes? A systematic review. Soc Sci Med 2010 May;70(9):1423–40. https://doi.org/10.1016/j.socscimed.2009.12.037.

[87] Reynolds AJ, Temple JA, Robertson DL, Mann EA. Long-term effects of an early childhood intervention on educational achievement and juvenile arrest: a 15-year follow-up of low-income children in public schools. JAMA 2001 May;285(18):2339–46. https://doi.org/10.1001/jama.285.18.2339.

[88] Tandon PS, Zhou C, Lozano P, Christakis DA. Preschoolers' total daily screen time at home and by type of child care. J Pediatr 2011 Feb;158(2):297–300. https://doi.org/10.1016/j.jpeds.2010.08.005.

[89] Webster EK, Martin CK, Staiano AE. Fundamental motor skills, screen-time, and physical activity in preschoolers. J Sport Health Sci 2019 Mar;8(2):114–21. https://doi.org/10.1016/j.jshs.2018.11.006.

[90] Cox R, Skouteris H, Rutherford L, Fuller-Tyszkiewicz M, Dell'Aquila D, Hardy LL. Television viewing, television content, food intake, physical activity and body mass index: a cross-sectional study of preschool children aged 2–6 years. Health Promot J Austr 2012;23(1):58–62. https://doi.org/10.1071/HE12058.

[91] Suglia SF, Duarte CS, Chambers EC, Boynton-Jarrett R. Social and behavioral risk factors for obesity in early childhood. J Dev Behav Pediatr 2013 Oct;34(8):549–56. https://doi.org/10.1097/DBP.0b013e3182a509c0.

[92] Dennison BA, Erb TA, Jenkins PL. Television viewing and television in bedroom associated with overweight risk among low-income preschool children. Pediatrics 2002 Jun;109(6):1028–35. https://doi.org/10.1542/peds.109.6.1028.

[93] Goncalves WSF, Byrne R, Viana MT, Trost SG. Parental influences on screen time and weight status among preschool children from Brazil: a cross-sectional study. Int J Behav Nutr Phys Act 2019 Mar;16. https://doi.org/10.1186/s12966-019-0788-3.

[94] Pearson N, Biddle SJH. Sedentary behavior and dietary intake in children, adolescents, and adults. A systematic review. Am J Prev Med 2011 Aug;41(2):178–88. https://doi.org/10.1016/j.amepre.2011.05.002.

[95] Leech RM, McNaughton SA, Timperio A. The clustering of diet, physical activity and sedentary behavior in children and adolescents: a review. Int J Behav Nutr Phys Act 2014 Jan;11:4. https://doi.org/10.1186/1479-5868-11-4.

[96] Pearson N, Griffiths P, Biddle SJ, Johnston JP, McGeorge S, Haycraft E. Clustering and correlates of screen-time and eating behaviours among young adolescents. BMC Public Health 2017;17(1):533. https://doi.org/10.1186/s12889-017-4441-2.

[97] Russell SJ, Croker H, Viner RM. The effect of screen advertising on children's dietary intake: a systematic review and meta-analysis. Obes Rev 2019;20(4):554–68. https://doi.org/10.1111/obr.12812.

[98] Temple JL, Giacomelli AM, Kent KM, Roemmich JN, Epstein LH. Television watching increases motivated responding for food and energy intake in children. Am J Clin Nutr 2007 Feb;85(2):355–61. https://doi.org/10.1093/ajcn/85.2.355.

[99] Kunkel D, Mastro D, Ortiz M, McKinley C. Food marketing to children on U.S. Spanish-language television. J Health Commun 2013;18(9):1084–96. https://doi.org/10.1080/10810730.2013.768732.

[100] Taveras EM, Hohman KH, Price S, Gortmaker SL, Sonneville K. Televisions in the bedrooms of racial/ethnic minority children: how did they get there and how do we get them out? Clin Pediatr (Phila) 2009 Sep;48(7):715–9. https://doi.org/10.1177/0009922809335667.

[101] Frisvold DE. Head start participation and childhood obesity. SSRN Electron. J; 2006. https://doi.org/10.2139/ssrn.887433.

[102] Zhai F. Effects of head start on the outcomes of participants [Dissertation 3299311]. Ann Arbor: Columbia University; 2008.

[103] US Department of Health and Human Services. Physical Activity Guidelines for Americans. 2nd ed. Washington, DC: US Department of Health and Human Services; 2018.

[104] Moore SC, et al. Leisure time physical activity of moderate to vigorous intensity and mortality: a large pooled cohort analysis. PLoS Med 2012 Nov;9(11). https://doi.org/10.1371/journal.pmed.1001335.

[105] 2017–2018 National Survey of Children's Health (NSCH) data query, Data Resource Center for Child and Adolescent Health supported by Cooperative Agreement U59MC27866 from the US Department of Health and Human Services, Health Resources and Services Administration's Maternal and Child Health Bureau (HRSA MCHB).

[106] Gordon-Larsen P, McMurray RG, Popkin BM. Adolescent physical activity and inactivity vary by ethnicity: The National Longitudinal Study of Adolescent Health. J Pediatr 1999 Sep;135(3):301–6. https://doi.org/10.1016/S0022-3476(99)70124-1.

[107] Dowda M, Ainsworth BE, Addy CL, Saunders R, Riner W. Environmental influences, physical activity, and weight status in 8- to 16-year-olds. Arch Pediatr Adolesc Med 2001 Jun;155 (6):711. https://doi.org/10.1001/archpedi.155.6.711.

[108] Abbott RA, Davies PSW. Habitual physical activity and physical activity intensity: their relation to body composition in 5.0–10.5-y-old children. Eur J Clin Nutr 2004 Feb;58(2):285–91. https://doi.org/10.1038/sj.ejcn.1601780.

[109] Trost SG, Sirard JR, Dowda M, Pfeiffer KA, Pate RR. Physical activity in overweight and nonoverweight preschool children. Int J Obes (Lond) 2003 Jul;27(7):834–9. https://doi.org/10.1038/sj.ijo.0802311.

[110] Berkey CS, Rockett HRH, Gillman MW, Colditz GA. One-year changes in activity and in inactivity among 10- to 15-year-old boys and girls: relationship to change in body mass index. Pediatrics 2003 Apr;111(4):836–43. https://doi.org/10.1542/peds.111.4.836.

[111] Flores G, Maldonado J, Durán P. Making tortillas without lard: Latino parents' perspectives on healthy eating, physical activity, and weight-management strategies for overweight Latino children. J Acad Nutr Diet 2012 Jan;112(1):81–9. https://doi.org/10.1016/j.jada.2011.08.041.

[112] Slater SJ, Ewing R, Powell LM, Chaloupka FJ, Johnston LD, O'Malley PM. The association between community physical activity settings and youth physical activity, obesity, and body mass index. J Adolesc Health 2010 Nov;47(5):496–503. https://doi.org/10.1016/j.jadohealth.2010.03.017.

[113] Nguyen-Rodriguez ST, McClain AD, Spruijt-Metz D. Anxiety mediates the relationship between sleep onset latency and emotional eating in minority children. Eat Behav 2010 Dec;11(4):297–300. https://doi.org/10.1016/j.eatbeh.2010.07.003.

[114] Lumeng JC, Somashekar D, Appugliese D, Kaciroti N, Corwyn RF, Bradley RH. Shorter sleep duration is associated with increased risk for being overweight at ages 9 to 12 years. Pediatrics 2007 Nov;120(5):1020–9. https://doi.org/10.1542/peds.2006-3295.

[115] Seegers V, et al. Short sleep duration and body mass index: a prospective longitudinal study in preadolescence. Am J Epidemiol 2011 Mar;173(6):621–9. https://doi.org/10.1093/aje/kwq389.

[116] Wong WW, et al. Sleep duration of underserved minority children in a cross-sectional study. BMC Public Health 2013 Jul;13:648. https://doi.org/10.1186/1471-2458-13-648.

[117] Padez C, Mourao I, Moreira P, Rosado V. Long sleep duration and childhood overweight/obesity and body fat. Am J Hum Biol 2009 Jun;21(3):371–6. https://doi.org/10.1002/ajhb.20884.

[118] Katare B, Chakrovorty S. Association between environmental factors and BMI: evidence from recent immigrants from developing countries. J Health Popul Nutr 2019 Jul;38. https://doi.org/10.1186/s41043-019-0174-4.

[119] Antecol H, Bedard K. Unhealthy assimilation: why do immigrants converge to American health status levels? Demography 2006 May;43(2):337–60. https://doi.org/10.1353/dem.2006.0011.

[120] Himmelgreen DA, et al. The longer you stay, the bigger you get: length of time and language use in the U.S. are associated with obesity in Puerto Rican women. Am J Phys Anthropol 2004;125(1):90–6. https://doi.org/10.1002/ajpa.10367.

[121] McDonald JT, Kennedy S. Is migration to Canada associated with unhealthy weight gain? Overweight and obesity among Canada's immigrants. Soc Sci Med 2005 Dec;61(12): 2469–81. https://doi.org/10.1016/j.socscimed.2005.05.004.

Chapter 11

Cultural factors related to the obesity epidemic

Zohra Salehi, M.D., Pharm.D.
Hospital Medicine, Hartford HealthCare, Hartford, CT, United States

Introduction

The prevalence of obesity is known to vary according to socioculture factors. Additionally, patterns can be specific to race, age, and gender with relationships observed in developed countries. Culture is defined as a social construct, an idea created and accepted by society formed by norms, values, and beliefs; culture is usually taught and passed down from one generation to the next. Ethnicity is a form of cultural identity where a social group belongs to a common culture. Race, on the other hand, is commonly mistaken with ethnicity but is in fact biologically based and needs a more universal definition to be used in the medical literature [1]. The US Census Bureau categorizes race as American Indian or Alaska Native, Asian, Black or African American, Native Hawaiian or other Pacific Islander, and White. Ethnicity is categorized as Hispanic or Latino (a person of Cuban, Mexican, Puerto Rican, South or Central American, or other Spanish culture or origin, regardless of race) and not Hispanic or Latino.

The obesity epidemic

Obesity is a preventable illness that is sweeping the globe with immensely high rates found in the United States. Although diet and exercise are commonly thought to be the basis for maintaining a healthy weight and lifestyle, obesity rates tend to vary across different demographics. Specifically, depending on gender, socioeconomic status, and ethnicity, there will be completely different rates of obesity within those subgroups, regardless of the national average [2]. Accordingly, clinical research is becoming more focused on the more nuanced trends that people see within more specialized sample sizes of people.

Because simple diet and exercise habits are not reducing the occurrence of obesity, scientists have to look deeper into the problem to quell the global public health concern. Prevention and control are the ideals, but to understand how to

Obesity. https://doi.org/10.1016/B978-0-12-818839-2.00011-9

prevent obesity from becoming an issue, people have to understand how and why it occurs in some people but not in others. The difference in obesity rates across race and ethnicity, age group, and gender are all leading clinicians to believe that the way to approach this problem is through epidemiological studies that look at obesity as a spreading disease rather than a preventable condition [2].

The influences of culture

Cultural and economic factors play a role in why some groups are more likely to be obese or overweight. In certain parts of the world, people who share a cultural background tend to reside in close proximity and have the same obesity risk, which can sometimes explain the trends in BMI. Food is an important part of different cultures and with migration to other countries, traditional cooking is passed forward. This explains why certain cultures, although in different countries, have the same obesity rates. This also indicates that food provides a physical link that connects individuals to their heritage, culture, and local communities [3]. Food is a way for identity maintenance and formation, connecting individuals to their heritage. It also serves as a tool for examining the degree to which immigrants are maintaining their cultural identity. Eating foods is culturally patterned and obesity can be influenced by the national culture of a population. Investigating the relationship between national culture and BMI has been performed by Masood et al. [4]. The study was performed to analyze the captured data from the World Health Survey (WHS) conducted in 2002–2004 by the World Health Organization (WHO) in 70 countries. The study included adults aged 18 years living in private households, but only 53 countries were included in the final study results [4]. Individual-level BMI was estimated by using height and weight, and factors included in the analysis were sex, age, marital status, education, occupation, economic status, and location. The study found that there is a positive association between age and BMI, with a 0.34 unit increase for every 10 years increase in age. BMI for married groups was higher than in nonmarried groups; wealthier quintiles had higher BMI than the lowest quintile.

Hofstede's cultural dimensions theory on society and obesity

Hofstede, a renowned psychologist, developed a cultural dimension theory and described cultures across different dimensions, including power distance, individualism, uncertainty avoidance, and masculinity. Hofstede's cultural dimension theory on society and obesity can help us to better understand how, for example, cultures are influenced by ambiguity, uncertainty, risks, etc. High uncertainty avoidance cultures are defined as those that live in a society where their culture is in line with careful planning to reduce risks by attempting to control future events. Countries that fall under the high-risk uncertainty avoidance index are Russia, Italy, and Korea. Countries with low uncertainty avoidance index countries are the United Kingdom, the United States, and China. Those living in a high uncertainty avoidance culture were found to have a positive association with BMI, and despite careful planning and structured rules and norms, their focus was more on the treatment of obesity rather than the prevention of overweight [4]. Other reasons for this inverse relationship are tolerance to risks and challenges to instill ownership of obesity prevention. In cultures with a high uncertainty avoidance index, people expect health professionals to provide solutions [5, 6], with curative rather preventive attitudes in people toward obesity. People in high uncertainty avoidance societies find difficulty accepting recommendations to prevent obesity, so this factor must be taken into account when designing a public policy that aims to target obesity intervention plans. Proposed concepts to aid in better policymaking in high avoidance uncertainty index countries are using facts and statistics, decreasing elements of the unknown, and providing enough time to help improve understanding [7, 8]. Uncertainty avoidance and individualism (UAI) societies (e.g., Canada and the United States) were significantly associated with BMI, showing that people in more individualistic or high uncertainty avoidance countries had higher BMIs than collectivist or low uncertainty avoidance ones. The collectivist societies (e.g., China, Japan, India) believe that health is controlled by external sources beyond their control such as family and society. In collectivist societies, families tend to eat together, portion sizes are reduced, and snacking behavior is less frequent [7, 9, 10]. Thus, the culture of collectivist society will likely implement eating patterns on specific mealtimes, proportions, and the types of foods being consumed.

Eating patterns of cultures

Cultural patterns of eating can be influenced by cultural views of health and wellness as well as the frequency and size of the meal. For example, energy intake is influenced by the sociocultural context of how many people are eating a meal together. Ideas about health can be cultural and can vary with each society.

Patterns of eating can be influenced by cultural views of health and wellness, including the frequency, portion, and size of the meal. Determining meal portions and consequently the energy intake, one can be influenced by how many people one is eating with [11]. Eating with one other person increases the average amount of food ingested in meals by 44% compared to easting alone, and meals eaten in large groups were up to 75% larger than when eaten alone [11]. The types of foods consumed are based on what the culture finds appealing and acceptable to consume [11].

Mediterranean regions

The Mediterranean diets are characterized by a high intake of vegetables, fruits, nuts, cereals, whole grains, and olive oil; the moderate consumption of fish and poultry; and the low intake of sweets, red meat, and dairy products. This diet is proven to have many health benefits, including preventing obesity. However, with the change in globalization, many regions of Spain, Greece, and Italy are slowly opting out of this cultural healthy diet. Mediterranean countries are facing higher obesity rates and this could be associated with the higher consumption of fast foods and sodas instead of the traditional Mediterranean diet. This exemplifies that culture trends, the choice of foods, and the pattern of meals are linked to psychological and physical variables and that these are changing with time [11]. Another explanation for differences in eating habits among people from different regions is that they carry their own views of what well-being stands for and these views may stem from their migration, social practices, their own illnesses [12], and social networks. To bring about wellness in a society, one must take into account the objectivity of science and the subjectivity of culture for individual health maintenance [12].

Japan

The country with the lowest obesity rate is Japan with <4% of its population being obese. The Japanese traditional diet (Washoku) emphasizes smaller food portions, with an emphasis on rice, vegetables, steamed foods, soups with high water content, and less animal fat and sweets, to help maintain lower caloric intake [13]. The etiquette of eating and the Japanese culture foster enthusiasm and calmness during mealtimes with family and friends, which adds to the slower eating time and thereby increases the feeling of fullness that, in turn, makes them eat fewer portions [13]. The Japanese population eats on average 200 fewer calories than the recommended caloric intake. The socioeconomic factor with a high cost of transportation makes the population prone to increased physical activity and walking [13].

Pacific Islands

The Pacific region, also referred to as Oceania, consists of people that include Melanesians, Polynesians, Micronesians, Papuans, and indigenous Australians. This is a group of indigenous people with a certain burden of infectious and noncommunicable diseases. One of the greatest health problems facing the Pacific people of Polynesia is obesity [14]. In at least 10 Pacific island countries, more than 50% (and in some, up to 90%) of the population are overweight according to the WHO survey [15]. Although social and environmental factors such as poverty along with food shortage and accessibility to health care are factors that can affect wellness, the WHO reports that one of the main issues is the poor diet they consume. One of the biggest reasons for this is the replacement of traditional foods with imported foods that contain higher calories [15]. Other factors including genetics can also play a role. Recent developments in personalized medicine have shown that identifying ethnicity-linked genetic vulnerabilities can be important for medical management [16]. This is theorized to be because of the thrifty phenotype hypothesis, where “thrifty factors” are developed within the womb as a direct result of the environment in the womb. The theory is that insulin resistance is related to predicting the life of starvation for the fetus [17]. This thrifty factor is a mechanism to cope with food shortage and an adaptation could be factored in the development of obesity [14].

The Eastern Mediterranean region (Saudi Arabia, Lebanon, Bahrain)

This region is characterized by one of the highest burdens of overweight and obesity worldwide [18]. Of more concern is the high level of childhood obesity in countries in the region, with approximately 10% of school-aged children being obese, an estimate that is projected to follow an escalating trend [19]. The prevalence of overweight is highest among boys, with the highest rates at the age of 10–13 years and with a decline thereafter [18]. Among girls, the prevalence of overweight and obesity was the highest at 6–9 years, with the prevalence of elevated waist circumference reaching its highest in girls aged 14 and 17 years.

The relationship between demographic and socioeconomic factors and dietary/energy intake patterns differs in rural versus urban areas in the Middle East region of Lebanon. A multivariate study of 800 Lebanese school-aged children between the ages of 6–18 years was done during a time when Lebanon was going through a nutritional transition. The study showed that, as compared to subjects living in the capital (Beirut), those residing in other areas had a significantly lower odds ratio of being overweight. Obesity in rural versus urban populations could be explained by adopting the Western pattern of eating fast foods [20]. Overweight and obesity in the school-aged children were positively associated with a sedentary nature, irregular breakfast consumption, and the intake of fast food and sugary beverages. A healthier lifestyle such as eating milk/dairy and olive oil was associated with a lowered risk. As maternal education went up, this was found to be associated with higher odds of being overweight among the socioeconomic characteristics of those ages 6–11 while paternal education had a negative association. This study highlights the importance of culture, socioeconomic, and age differences in lifestyle and dietary habits [21].

Canada

The associations of sociodemographics, lifestyle, and food choice are factors that play a role in obesity. The Canadian Population Health Initiative found that social, environment, and individual factors can influence people’s eating habits and are independently related to obesity. In 2019, health data statistics showed

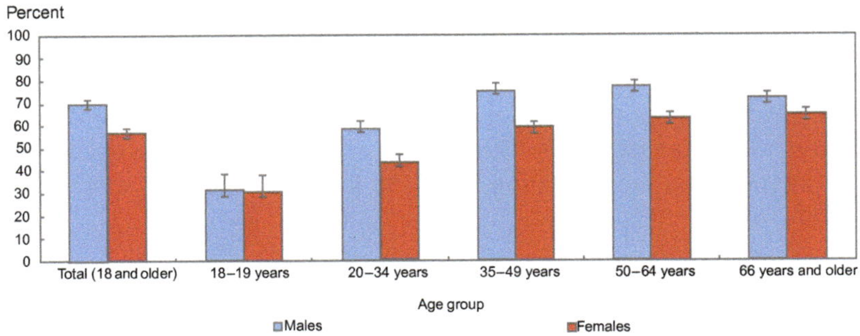

FIG. 1 Overweight or obese (adjusted), by age group and sex, population aged 18 and older, Canada, 2018. *(Source: Canadian Community Health Survey, 2018.)*

that 17.2 million Canadians were obese or overweight, comprising approximately 63.1% of the population. The proportion of adults who were obese decreased as education increased, from 34.5% among households where the highest level of education was less than secondary school graduation to 25.5% where at least one household member had completed postsecondary education (Fig. 1) [22].

In Canada, the high prevalence of obesity, with risks for health complications, has prompted more research for policy and monitoring. The factors associated with overweight were low literacy, low-income level, physical inactivity, and poor diet quality, such as less consumption of fruits and vegetables. Social inequality can serve as a determinant of health, especially in the vulnerable population [23].

Risk factors for obesity in adults in California

One might think that an obesity study on a sample size of people specifically from California would yield a collection of similar results. However, the disparities that we see between different ethnicities throughout the rest of the world also can be seen within a study done exclusively on Californians. In fact, California was selected specifically to examine how ethnic differences exist within an established average obesity rate. Because there are so many different races represented within California, scientists were able to see the result of a combination of American culture and ethnic obesity prevalence.

One of their key findings was the difference in overall obesity rates by ethnicity. African Americans (36%) and Latinos (33.6%) were far more likely to be diagnosed with obesity than Whites (22%) or Asians (9.8%) [24]. These observations suggest that there are factors that contribute to obesity prevalence beyond ethnicity, such as biological, sociocultural, and environmental factors (Table 1).

TABLE 1 Cultural factors related to the obesity epidemic.

Obesity prevalence in racial/ethnic minority populations vs. reference populations in the United States, Europe, Australia, and New Zealand.

Population and data source[a] and year	*Ethnic group*		
United States [19]		Males	Females
Data source: National Health and Nutrition Examination Survey, 2013–16	Non-Hispanic white	36.2 (33.1–39.5)	38.1 (35.6–40.6)
	Non-Hispanic black	37.4 (33.8–41.2)	55.9 (53.0–58.9)
% (95% CI) of adults ages 20 and older with BMI $\geq$30 kg/m^2, age adjusted	Hispanic	40.6 (36.5–44.7)	48.9 (45.3–52.4)
	Non-Hispanic Asian	11.2 (8.8–13.9)	13.6 (11.1–16.5)
United States [26]		Combined males and females	
Data source: National Health Interview Survey, 2016	Non-Hispanic white	28.7 (0.42)	
% (SE) of adults ages 18 years and older with BMI $\geq$30 kg/m^2, age adjusted, based on self-reported weight and height	Non-Hispanic black	39.4 (1.18)	
	Mexican American	34.1 (1.26)	
	American Indian or Alaska Native	39.1 (1.26)	
	Asian	9.54 (0.94)	
	Native Hawaiian/ Pacific Islander	51.7 (6.97)	
Canada [18]	Canada	16.9	
Data source: Canadian Community Health Survey, 2007–2008	Aboriginal (off-reserve)	25.7[b]	
% of adults ages 18 years and older with BMI $\geq$30 kg/m^2, based on self-reported weight and height			
Amsterdam, The Netherlands [25]	Dutch	10[c]	

Continued

TABLE 1 Cultural factors related to the obesity epidemic—cont'd

Obesity prevalence in racial/ethnic minority populations vs. reference populations in the United States, Europe, Australia, and New Zealand.

Population and data source and year	*Ethnic group*		
Data source: HELIUS Study Cohort, 2011–15	Turkish	35	
% of adults 18–70 years with BMI ≥30 kg/m^2	Moroccan	29	
	South Asian Surinamese	19	
	African Surinamese	30	
	Ghanaian	34	
England [21]		Males	Females
Data source: Health Survey for England, 2006–10 (average)	White	18.8	18.7
% of adults ages 16+ years with BMI > 30 kg/m^2, age standardized	Black Caribbean[e]	20.9	25.5
	Black African[d,e]	16.0	31.6
	Indian	13.2	13.1
	Pakistani[d,e]	12.2	26.2
	Bangladeshi	11.5	15.1
New Zealand [35]	European	28.6 (26.5–30.9)	32.2 (30.6–33.8)
Data source: New Zealand Health Survey, 2016–17	Maori	48.8 (44.6–53.0)	51.5 (48.5–54.5)
% (95% CI) of adults ages 15 years and older with BMI ≥30 kg/m^2, age adjusted	Pacific	63.6 (55.5–70.9)	73.4 (67.1–78.9)
	Asian	15.8 (12.4–20.0)	13.6 (10.8–17.1)
Australia [17][f]		Males	Females
Data sources: Australian Aboriginal and Torres Strait Islander Health Survey, 2012–13 and 2011–12, Australian Health Survey		Ages 35–44 years	

TABLE 1 Cultural factors related to the obesity epidemic—cont'd

Obesity prevalence in racial/ethnic minority populations vs. reference populations in the United States, Europe, Australia, and New Zealand.			
Population and data source and year	*Ethnic group*		
% of adults with BMI ≥30 kg/m^2 by age groups	Aboriginal and Torres Strait islander	43	50
	Nonindigenous	30	25
		Ages 45–54 years	
	Aboriginal and Torres Strait Islander[g]	35	49
	Nonindigenous	32	30
		Ages 55 and over	
	Aboriginal and Torres Strait islander	44	50
	Nonindigenous	35	32

[a]*Based on measured weight and height unless otherwise noted.*
[b]*Statistically different from nonaboriginal (P < .05).*
[c]*Source states that prevalence compared to Dutch is higher in the other ethnic groups.*
[d]*Prevalence is higher among women than men.*
[e]*Prevalence of obesity among women is higher than in other ethnic groups.*
[f]*Overall age-adjusted obesity prevalence for aboriginal and Torres Strait islander people ages 15 to 55+ was 1.5 times higher than in nonindigenous people—male ratio 1.4 and female ratio 1.7; age-specific rates shown were estimated from bar graphs in the source.*
[g]*Difference between aboriginal and Torres Strait islander rate and nonindigenous rate is not significant in this group; male female difference is significant in this age group.*
BMI, body mass index; CI, confidence interval; SE, standard error.
Kumanyika SK. Unraveling common threads in obesity risk among racial/ethnic minority and migrant populations. Public Health 2019; 172, 125–134. https://doi.org/10.1016/j.puhe.2019.04.010.

In addition, this study saw that physical activity did not necessarily prevent obesity in adults. Specifically, the study found that physical activity protected Whites and African Americans against obesity, but Hispanic/Latinos and Asians were less likely to see that same result, even if they met the recommendations for daily physical activity. The federal guidelines for activity recommend that adults do at least 150 min (2 h and 30 min) to 300 min (5 h) per week of moderate intensity. Whites were more likely to meet the federal guidelines than the Asian, African American, or Hispanic/Latino populations [24]. This suggests that while a good diet and exercise might be the basis for a healthy lifestyle, ethnicity and genetics might play a larger role than most people anticipated when it comes to maintaining a healthy weight. There are factors that people tend to be born with that might predispose them to an unhealthy weight, in spite of their best efforts.

The negative impact of sweetened beverages and skipping breakfast on obesity in children

Energy compensation is defined as the adjustment of energy intake provoked by the previous ingestion of a given stimulus (preload), whether if a snack or a beverage is consumed [25]. Insufficient energy compensation has been associated with increased energy intake and positive energy balance, leading to obesity [26, 27]. Thus, this implies that energy intake is significantly higher each day an energy-bearing beverage consumed, because of the insufficient energy compensation associated with the drink sweetened beverages with high sugar content.

Many studies have shown a connection between the consumption of sugar-sweetened beverages and total energy intake, where excess calories from the soda or calorically sweetened beverage can contribute to more weight gain through excess calories [9, 19, 28–30]. When children are substituting sweetened beverages and increasing their weight, the specific dietary habits impact the risk of obesity. The importance of not skipping breakfast in the study by Nasreddine et al. is well documented and finds that regular breakfast consumption was associated with a significantly lower risk of overweight and obesity. Skipping breakfast may lead to irregular eating habits as well as the consumption of higher amounts of calories at subsequent meals [31–33].

The impact of food types on weight gain in children: Fast foods versus dairies

The nutritional intake of foods has an impact on weight gain and the types of food intake among children and adolescents. In a study by Nasreddine et al., it was found that obesity was linked to age groups and the type of food intake. Adolescents aged 12–19 had a higher consumption of fast food and legumes and nuts, compared to children 6–11. The adolescent was also found to have higher energy/cal intakes, with their average energy intake being 2255.85 versus 1736.48 kcal/day (children). Children aged 6–11 did not consume as much fast food and were shown to have a higher intake of milk and dairy (8.90% vs. 6.47% in adolescents). Bread and cereals (36.92% vs. 32.67% adolescent) were significantly higher in children 6–11 compared to adolescents [21]. There was a negative association with higher intakes of milk and dairy products on the odds of obesity, and a positive association was documented between the higher consumption of sugar-sweetened beverages and overweight [21].

How social and environmental factors affect obesity

Environmental factors can include a number of different aspects of the place you live and the lifestyle you have. In terms of the United States, the Midwest and the South have the highest rates of obesity among adults. This can be attributed to the higher percentage of rural areas within those regions. Rural areas tend to have fewer convenient supermarkets, healthcare options, and activity-based recreation centers, which means residents of those areas have to work harder to fulfill healthy habits [34].

There is also the supply of healthy food to consider. Some areas are known for having very limited access to affordable and nutritious food. These areas are called "food deserts." A food desert can increase the likelihood that residents will have obesity by 30% [34]. Access to healthy food doesn't necessarily guarantee healthier lifestyles. In fact, when new grocery stores were introduced within food desert areas, BMI and the prevalence of obesity were not dramatically affected. Most people were just grateful to have access to healthier food. However, this doesn't mean that access to affordable healthy food is not important; it simply means that it is not the only important thing that contributes to overall health.

From a social perspective, some studies have shown that socioeconomic status has a major impact on overall health and obesity rates. Not only can people with more resources afford plenty of healthy, nutritious food, but their other needs are also being met effectively. This means that they have the stamina and the additional attention span necessary to prioritize a healthy lifestyle. Those who are focused on making sure they will be able to feed, clothe, and house their families often have priorities beyond health-focused goals [34]. And understandably so! Those who have disposable income and their basic needs met are people who can focus on creating healthy habits.

Hunger can also be psychological. Those who perceive themselves to be of a lower class or missing out on the privileges of a better life often tend to consume more high-calorie food versus those who perceive themselves as living a full life [34].

Conclusion

The purpose of this chapter was to determine if obesity is culturally influenced. Because culture is changing and people's beliefs are also being reshaped by society, the rise in obesity can partly be explained by culture but is in general multifactorial. First, race and ethnicity are linked to the prevalence of obesity, where we find obesity is more prevalent in Hispanics than non-Hispanics and Asians. Second, genetics can play a role in cultures with a high obesity rate.

Ethnically linked genetic variability is noted in Pacific Islanders where food is scarce, but obesity rates being among the highest in the world can be explained by changes in genetic inheritances although the importation of more high-calorie food. Third, Westernization has a major influence on changes in previously healthy culture eating habits. The Mediterranean countries of Greece, Italy, and Spain have noted an increase in obesity rates, partly due to a shift from Mediterranean foods to the consumption of Western foods (such as sodas and fast foods). This link of increased obesity to Western dietary patterns is also found among Eastern Mediterranean regions. The children in Lebanon who consumed more sodas, skipped breakfast, and ate more fast foods were shown to have higher patterns of obesity. Physical inactivity continues to be a major negative factor and is also a cause for why people gain weight globally. The only country with the lowest obesity rate is Japan, and the reason is due to more physical activity and healthier food choices in smaller portion sizes with a lower caloric intake, which is a cultural factor.

By understanding how and why certain areas and demographics are experiencing higher than average obesity levels, health professionals will be able to develop more effective preventative measures and reduce the rate of obesity and the diseases that come with it across the globe. When it comes to obesity prevention, knowledge is power. Products are constantly marketed as healthy choices by businesses, when in fact, they aren't healthy at all. It's the lack of transparency and the lack of education that leads people to make poor food choices. The end goal would be to implement early intervention programs and effective education that allows people to make more educated nutrition decisions. This would ultimately allow them to create effective health habits early enough in life that their weight does not pose a risk to their overall health. This leads directly to an analysis of the social and environmental factors that can have an effect on obesity rates within specific demographics.

References

[1] McKenzie KJ, Crowcroft NS. Race, ethnicity, culture, and science. BMJ 1994;309(6950): 286–7. https://doi.org/10.1136/bmj.309.6950.286.

[2] Arroyo-Johnson C, Mincey KD. Obesity epidemiology worldwide. Gastroenterol Clin North Am 2016 Dec;45(4):571–9. https://doi.org/10.1016/j.gtc.2016.07.012 PMID: 27837773; PMCID: PMC5599163.

[3] Weller DL, Turkon D. Contextualizing the immigrant experience: the role of food and foodways in identity maintenance and formation for first- and second-generation Latinos in Ithaca, New York. Ecol Food Nutr 2015;54(1):57–73.

[4] Masood M, Aggarwal A, Reidpath DD. Effect of national culture on BMI: a multilevel analysis of 53 countries. BMC Public Health 2019;19:1212. https://doi.org/10.1186/s12889-019-7536-0.

[5] Havold JI. National cultures and safety orientation: a study of seafarers working for Norwegian shipping companies. Work Stress 2007;21(2):173–95.

[6] Hofstede G. Dimensionalizing cultures: the Hofstede model in context. Online Readings in Psychology and Culture;2011:2(1).

[7] Hofstede G. Culture's consequences: comparing values, behaviors, institutions, and organizations across nations. 2nd ed. Thousand Oaks, CA: Sage Publications; 2001.

[8] Hofstede GH, Hofstede GJ. Cultures and organizations: software of the mind. New York; London: McGraw-Hill; 2005.

[9] Troiano RP, Briefel RR, Carroll MD, Bialostosky K. Energy and fat intakes of children and adolescents in the United States: data from the National Health and Nutrition Examination Surveys. Am J Clin Nutr 2000;72(Suppl):1343S–1353S.

[10] Vartanian LR, Herman CP, Wansink B. Are we aware of the externa3l factors that influence our food intake? Health Psychol 2008;27(5):533–8.

[11] De Castro J. Socio-cultural determinants of meal size and frequency. Br J Nutr 1997;77(S1): S39–55. https://doi.org/10.1079/BJN19970103.

[12] Napier AD, et al., Culture and health. Lancet 2014;384(9954):1607–39. https://doi.org/10.1016/S0140-6736(14)61603-2.

[13] Shubrook N. Why is the Japanese diet so healthy? https://www.bbcgoodfood.com/howto/guide/why-japanese-diet-so-healthy [Accessed 13 February 2020].

[14] NEEL JV. Diabetes mellitus: a 'Thrifty' genotype rendered detrimental by 'progress'? Am J Hum Genet 1962 Dec;14(4):353–62. www.ncbi.nlm.nih.gov/pmc/articles/PMC1932342/.

[15] World Health Organization. Bulletin of the World Health Organization. Vol. 88, No. 7, 2010 Jul. p. 481–560.

[16] Horwood PF, et al., Health challenges of the Pacific Region: insights from history, geography, social determinants, genetics, and the microbiome. Front Immunol 2019;10:2184. https://doi.org/10.3389/fimmu.2019.02184.

[17] Watve MG, Yajnik CS. Evolutionary origins of insulin resistance: a behavioral switch hypothesis. BMC Evol Biol 2007 Apr;7:61. www.ncbi.nlm.nih.gov/pmc/articles/PMC1868084/.

[18] Mehio S, Nasreddine L, Mokdad A, et al., Nutrition transition and cardiovascular disease risk factors in Middle East and North Africa countries: reviewing the evidence. Ann Nutr Metab 2010;57:193–203.

[19] Wang Y, Lobstein T. Worldwide trends in childhood overweight and obesity. Int J Pediatr Obes 2006;1:11–25, www.ncbi.nlm.nih.gov/pubmed/17902211.

[20] Hales CM, Carroll MD, Fryar CD, Ogden CL. Prevalence of obesity among adults and youth: United States, 2015–2016. NCHS Data Brief 2017;(288).

[21] Nasreddine L, et al., Dietary, lifestyle and socio-economic correlates of overweight, obesity and central adiposity in Lebanese children and adolescents. Nutrients 2014 Mar;63: 1038–62. https://doi.org/10.3390/nu6031038.

[22] Statistics Canada. Overweight and Obese Adults 2018. Chart 1: Overweight or obese (adjusted), by age group and sex, population aged 18 and older, Canada, 2018. Catalogue no.82-625-X; 2019. https://www150.statcan.gc.ca/n1/en/pub/82-625-x/2019001/article/00005-eng.pdf?st=GQJi3vI5. Accessed 17 February 2020.

[23] Socio-Demographic and Lifestyle Correlates of Obesity. Cora Lynn Craig, Canadian Fitness and Lifestyle Research Institute (CFLRI), Christine Cameron (CFLRI) and Adrian Bauman (University of New South Wales/CFLRI). https://secure.cihi.ca/free_products/Sociodemographic_Lifestyle_e.pdf. [Accessed 30 January 2020].

[24] Wang L, Southerland J, Wang K, Bailey BA, Alamian A, Stevens MA, et al., Ethnic differences in risk factors for obesity among adults in California, the United States. J Obes 2017;2017. 2427483. Available from: https://www.ncbi.nlm.nih.gov/pmc/articles/PMC5352906/.

[25] Blundell J, et al., Appetite control: methodological aspects of the evaluation of foods. Obes Rev Feb. 2010;11(3):251–70. https://doi.org/10.1111/j.1467789x.2010.00714.

[26] Almiron-Roig E, Chen Y, Drewnowski A. Liquid calories and the failure of satiety: how good is the evidence? Obes Rev 2003;4:201–12.

[27] Jebb SA, Siervo M, Fruhbeck G, et al., Variability of appetite control mechanisms in response to 9 weeks of progressive overfeeding in humans. Int J Obes (Lond) 2006;30:1160–2.

[28] Anand R, Basiotis P. Is total fat consumption really decreasing? Washington, DC: USDA Center for Nutrition Policy and Promotion; 1998 [Nutrition Insights 5].

[29] Berkey CS, Rockett HR, Field AE, Gillman MW, Colditz GA. Sugar-added beverages and adolescent weight change. Obes Res 2004;12:778–88 [PubMed: 15166298].

[30] Johnson RK, Frary C. Choose beverages and foods to moderate your intake of sugars: the 2000 Dietary Guidelines for Americans—what's all the fuss about? J Nutr 2001;131:2766S–71S.

[31] Deshmukh-Taskar PR, Radcliffe JD, Liu Y, Nicklas TA. Do breakfast skipping and breakfast type affect energy intake, nutrient intake, nutrient adequacy, and diet quality in young adults? NHANES 1999–2002. J Am Coll Nutr 2010;29:407–18.

[32] Szajewska H, Ruszczyński M. Systematic review demonstrating that breakfast consumption influences body weight outcomes in children and adolescents in Europe. Crit Rev Food Sci Nutr 2010;50(2):113–9. https://doi.org/10.1080/10408390903467514.

[33] Lioret S, Volatier JL, Lafay L, Touvier M, Maire B. Is food portion size a risk factor of childhood overweight? Eur J Clin Nutr 2009;63:382–91.

[34] Lee A, Cardel M, Donahoo WT. Social and environmental factors influencing obesity. In: Feingold KR, Anawalt B, Boyce A, et al., editors. Endotext. South Dartmouth, MA: MDText.com, Inc.; 2000. Available from: https://www.ncbi.nlm.nih.gov/books/NBK278977/.

[35] Euler R, Jimenez EY, Sanders S, Kuhlemeier A, Van Horn ML, Cohen D, et al., Rural–urban differences in baseline dietary intake and physical activity levels of adolescents. Prev Chronic Dis 2019;16:180200. https://doi.org/10.5888/pcd16.180200.

Further reading

Ogden CL, Fakhouri TH, Carroll MD, et al., Prevalence of obesity among adults, by household income and education—United States, 2011–2014. Morb Mortal Wkly Rep 2017; 66:1369–73. https://doi.org/10.15585/mmwr.mm6650a1External.

de Vijver FJR V, van Hemert DA, Ype H. Multilevel analysis of individuals and cultures. New York; London: Psychology; 2008.

Chapter 12

Educational factors related to the obesity epidemic

Zohra Salehi, M.D., Pharm.D.
Hospital Medicine, Hartford HealthCare, Hartford, CT, United States

Introduction

Education can be used as an indicator of socioeconomic positions and also as an indicator of future health patterns. Educational attainment can be measured as the highest level of education that an individual has completed. Literacy is defined by the ability to read and write, and the average number of years spent in school (duration of each level of education). This chapter will focus on the educational factors that are related to the obesity trend.

Education attainment statistics

World statistic trends show that the average number of years spent in school has increased, given the expansion of education since the 19th century. Increased number of years of total schooling, as shown in Fig. 1, is a strong indicator that individuals within society are appreciating the value of education. The world population size by the education level of the secondary and tertiary school is larger and predicted to be higher by 2100. Three-fourths of countries are also increasing education spending as a share of the GDP. Global literacy is another measure of education and current data show that there are larger fractions of the population that are literate rather than illiterate (Fig. 2). For example, in 2016, the literate world population versus illiterate was 86.02% and 13.98%, respectively [1].

Literacy continues to rise in younger generations, reducing inequalities in the ability to read and write in the global population. It is projected that by 2050, only five countries in the world will have a population with a rate of no formal education above 20%: Burkina Faso, Ethiopia, Guinea, Mali, and Nigerno [2]. As countries develop over time, the share of population with no formal education, as displayed in Fig. 3, is predicted to decrease with time.

Obesity. https://doi.org/10.1016/B978-0-12-818839-2.00012-0

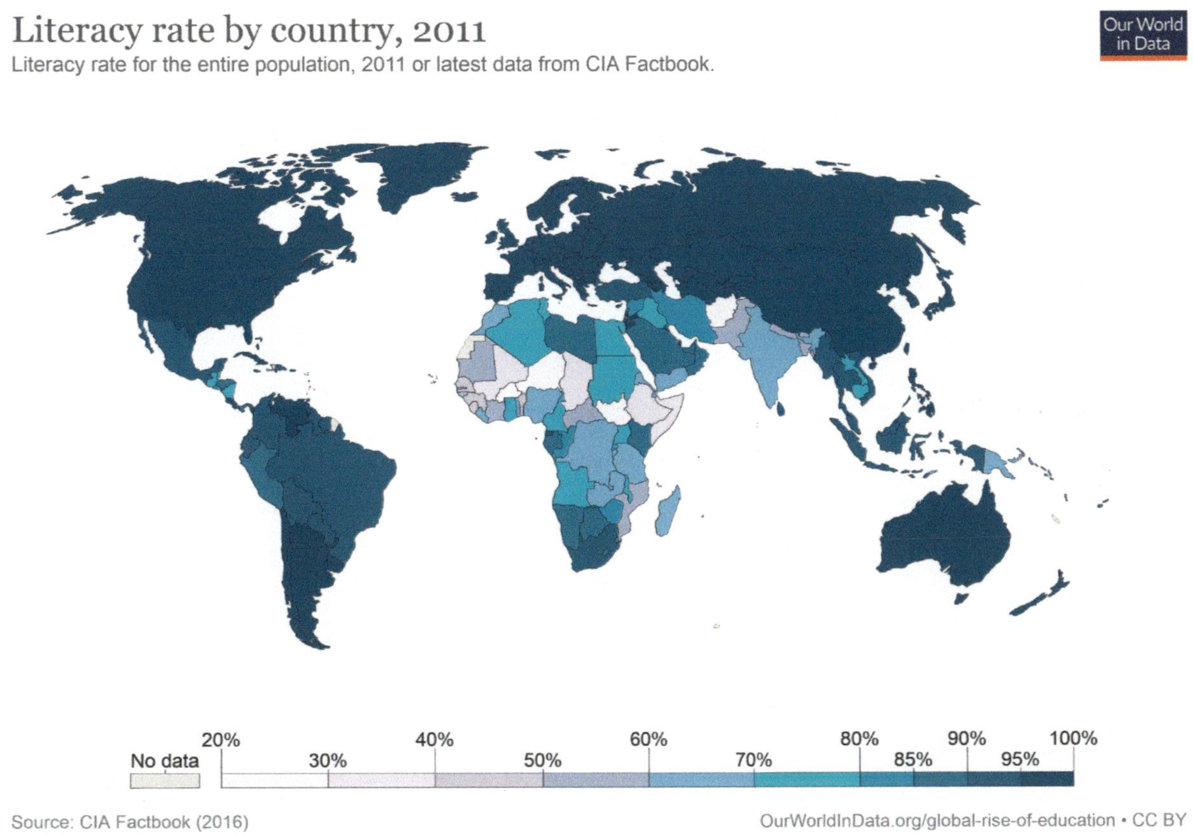

FIG. 1 Literacy distribution globally. *(Reprinted from Roser M, Ortiz-Ospina E. Global education. Our World in Data; 2016 Aug. http://ourworldindata.org/global-education. [Accessed 13 February 2020].)*

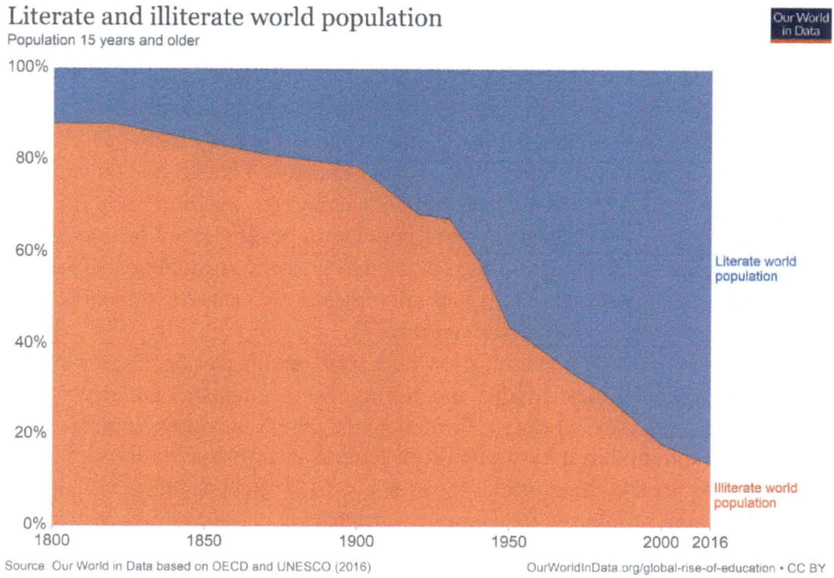

FIG. 2 Growing literacy in the last two centuries. *(Reprinted from Roser M, Ortiz-Ospina E. Global education. Our World in Data; 2016 Aug. http://ourworldindata.org/global-education. [Accessed 13 February 2020].)*

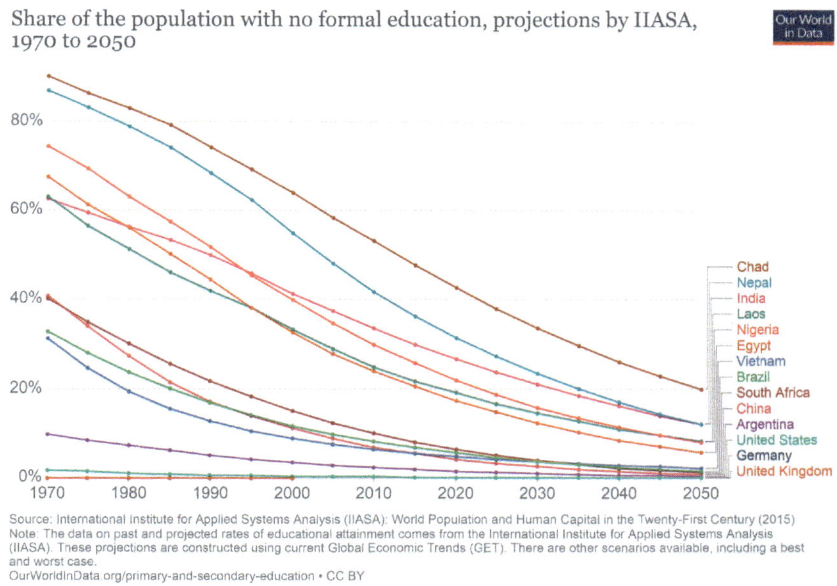

FIG. 3 The rate of education increases as the world develops. *(Reprinted from Roser M, Ortiz-Ospina E. Global education. Our World in Data; 2016 Aug. http://ourworldindata.org/global-education. [Accessed 13 February 2020])*

As more and more people gain literacy, the rate of no education is expected to close the cross country gaps. United States and China that currently have a rate of no formal education above 20%, is projected to only have a rate of 0.05% and 0.81%, respectively, by 2050 (Fig. 3). The current projection data support the assumption that cross-country gaps in literacy may close by 2050 [2].

Educational attainment can be used as an indicator of health outcomes in developed countries and as an indicator of socioeconomic position as well [3, 4]. Social class is also a key determinant of population health. Social inequalities in health are rising in the United States alongside growing inequalities in income and wealth. Conversely, research and surveillance to measure socioeconomic positions in health research are seldom met [3].

The association of poor education and poor health has been consistently observed in many studies. Studies examining the mechanisms underlying this association have looked at only a limited set of potential routes. Improvement in education attainment may transmit to general improvements in population health and the need to target specific pathways [5]. Tying education with health has been an area of interest for numerous studies, as certain interventions may improve education. For example, studies have found that other methods of improving education outside of socioeconomic status are introducing new policy changes targeting health literacy and health behaviors [5].

According to a host of research studies, the direct correlation of socioeconomic status with obesity and weight change varies with reporting findings [6]. Previous studies looking at the relationship between SES and obesity, by Sobal and Stunkard in 1989 [9], found in 144 published articles from the 1960s to the mid-1980s an inverse correlation for women in developed societies with a higher likelihood of obesity in those with low SES, and with inconsistent relations for men and children in developed countries [7]. The variable factor from 144 published articles was that according to Sobal and Stunkard, the articles did not specifically set out to study the association of SES with obesity but investigated the association in the course of examining other issues.

Income inequality as a health concern

During the 1970s, income inequality in the United States began to increase after narrowing considerably in the 1960s, and then it rose sharply in the 1980s [8]. Monitoring the inequalities in health requires obtaining data on population health. Our understanding of what the socioeconomic parameters are will help us to understand why it's important to measure socioeconomic conditions.

Body size and socioeconomic status

Building upon the work by Soba et al., a 2007 cross-sectional study by McLaren reviewed a total of 333 published articles between 1998 and 2004, and determined a relationship between SES and obesity. The results for both men and women had a positive association (high SES was associated with smaller body size) in countries with high levels of socioeconomic development. The opposite was true for areas with a low level of development. The study found variations in association depending on SES indicators. A negative association (low SES and large body size) in highly developed countries among women was most common with education and occupation. Conversely, in medium- and low-development countries, positive associations in women were common with income and material possessions [7].

The results of 333 published studies point to transitionary changes in the association as one moves from high human development index (HDI) countries to medium/low HDI countries. HDI assigned by the United Nations Development Program characterizes and ranks countries on a number of attributes, including life expectancy at birth, school enrollment, adult literacy, and standard of living based on the gross domestic product. Examples of HDI countries are Norway, the United Kingdom, and Germany (high); Brazil, Columbia, and Saudi Arabia (medium); and Cameroon, Benin, and Zambia (low). The study performed by McLaren confirmed negative associations (lower SES associated with larger body size) seen in women in high HDI countries, with a 63% negative association found. This negative effect is prominent for the following SES indicators: education, 72% negative; area-level indicators, 71% negative; occupation, 68% negative; and composite indicators, 67% negative. However, as one moved from high to medium to low HDI status, the proportion of positive associations (low SES associated with smaller body size) increased to 43% in medium-HDI countries and to 94% in low-HDI countries [7]. The highlights of the review analysis by McLaren display the role of economics on obesity in the developing world. Countries with a lower food supply and a lower cost for food can explain the negative associations in low-HDI countries. Furthermore, in low-HDI countries, the culture sometimes values a larger body weight, helping to explain the positive associations with larger body sizes [9].

To further answer the hypothesis of whether any relationship between education and obesity exists, a widened search of preexisting articles mostly through cross-sectional data, including more databases and languages, was performed by Cohen et al. Peer-reviewed articles between 1977 and 2012 looked at an individual's own educational status, with variations in weight and educational attainment. The relationships between education and obesity were classified as directly associated (as education increases, so do the odds or risks of obesity), inversely associated (as education decreases, the odds or risks of obesity increase), and null (no statistically significant relationship.). Education was measured as years of schooling and achievement. Weight was defined by BMI, with obesity defined as BMI >30 as well as measures of skin-fold thickness and waist-hip ratio.

The conclusion from the review study found a relationship between socioeconomic status, educational attainment, and obesity, depending on the country's level of development [1]. Inverse associations were more common in more-developed countries, meaning that as education decreases, obesity increases; positive associations were more common in less-developed countries. Further studies are needed to explore additional covariates in making associations between obesity and education [1].

Finding an association between modifiable risk factors and obesity among high school students in the United States was studied and analyzed by the US Department of Health in 2018. A retrospective study with a weighted sample of 15,624 respondents—7955 (51.3%) boys and 7551 (48.7%) girls—was performed. The demographics were non-Hispanic white (54.5%), Hispanic (22.3%), and black (13.6%). Among all respondents, 2005 (13.9%) had obesity. A greater proportion of boys (16.8%) than girls (10.8%) had obesity. A significant proportion of high school students engaged in unhealthy dietary, physical activity, or other lifestyle behaviors was also examined. About 24.7% of students watched television for 3h or more per day on an average school day; sports activity involvement found that 42.4% did not play on any sports team during the past school year. Understanding the lifestyle behaviors, the study showed that several unhealthy behaviors such as watching television for 3h or more per day, not sleeping more than 8h a day, smoking, and not participating in sports were modifiable risk factors for obesity that can be targeted as areas for more education and intervention [10].

The role of education in obesity

Aside from having one's own educational status to determine a correlation with obesity, educating people is a factor that can directly measure the impact of the obesity trend. One example is the role of intense lifestyle modification over 6months among overweight and obese subjects. The goal of this study was to achieve a mean loss of 5–10% of the baseline weight, reducing caloric intake by 500–1000kcal per day, and modifying dietary therapy with a diet encompassing fruits, vegetables, low-fat items, low-fat dairy and grain, and high fibers. Daily activity modification included changes in lifestyle such as walking rather than riding and using stairs rather than elevators. It was recommended that participants increase their physical activity to 3–5 times a week. The subjects were given education on behavior changes related to weight loss and how to record these changes. Lifestyle counseling was also delivered in sessions by a specialist in nutrition.

The subjects of the trial were 81 females (58%) and 59 males (42%), with a BMI of 30 ± 0.2. The study found statistically significant weight loss in both men and women at the end of 3 and 6months. The mean weight loss at the end of 3 and 6months was 3.7 ± 0.15 and 7.6 ± 0.8 kg compared with baseline weight, respectively ($P < 0.001$ and 0.001). Medication such as orlistat given to 30 subjects showed added benefits in weight loss; however, some participants did not tolerate its side effects. The mean weight loss in the orlistat group was 9.3 ± 1.8 kg ($P < .001$) compared with the baseline weight. The study concluded that 10% weight loss is achievable over a 6-month period with education about lifestyle, physical activity, and dietary modification as well as additional benefits with medication, orlistat, and counseling [11].

Educational attainment and obesity

Although education has proven to be a factor in obesity prevention and early intervention, the system is not perfect. In fact, an in-depth look at the literature designed to study the relationship between education and obesity shows that the literature often fails to take into account race and ethnicity as factors [1]. While it is certainly true that gender, age, and geography are factors that need to be taken into account, race and ethnicity are also critical points to consider when studying the correlation between obesity and other potential contributing factors. Our biological background does make a difference when it comes to health risk factors, and obesity is no different. Doctors and health care professionals need to look at their patients' comprehensive background to understand exactly what their patients need to be healthy and to combat obesity.

Unfortunately, it's only recently that obesity has begun to be looked at as an epidemic rather than simply a preventable disease that people need to fix for themselves. In fact, in a study evaluating the quality of articles designed to educate the public about obesity, only 10% of the 289 that were evaluated met the criteria for being considered a quality source [1]. It was only in more recent studies done in 2005 or later that higher-quality research was executed, and more factors were taken into account.

Science's understanding of obesity and the factors that contribute to a rise in weight gain are evolving with time. Studies are now being done to more fully understand the influence of factors such as socioeconomic position, geography, and education levels, and fortunately, it's becoming more common for scientists to look at participants of these studies more closely and evaluate their full demographic classification, rather than just their age and gender [1].

These studies have also started to investigate how social influences can play a role in higher obesity rates. The environment in which you live and grow up naturally has a bearing on people's overall health habits. There are a number of solutions that could be implemented to introduce an environment where healthy eating habits are fostered early in life. This could involve introducing more effective education within the school system or instituting policies for developing healthier habits among the students. Although obesity has historically been considered to be a wholly preventable disease, the dramatic rise in obesity rates in recent decades has forced health professionals to consider that other factors are playing a huge role in society's overall health while diet and exercise are the basis for maintaining a healthy weight and lifestyle.

Relationship between health literacy and obesity

The role of literacy skills may play a role in obesity risk. The prevalence of obesity was studied in Iran, a developing country in the Middle East. The prevalence of obesity in educational levels in Iranian adults was studied in a cross-sectional descriptive study based on population and 2452 cases (1224 men and 1228 women) aged 15–65 years [12]. In northern Iranian adults, the level of education defined as years of schooling and urbanization had an implication on obesity risk. The study found that the risk of obesity was 2.294 ($P = .001$) in the uneducated compared to high school or college-educated people, 1.668 ($P = .001$). In urban areas compared to rural areas, the risk of obesity was 2.044 ($P = .001$) in uneducated people compared to high school or college-educated subjects [12]. Uneducated adults had a higher prevalence than uneducated subjects below the age of 40. Moreover, the results found the prevalence of obesity in people aged 40–65 was 6.7% more than in people aged 15–40 years ($P = .234$) [12]. Obesity has a negative association with lower education levels and intervention to tackle educating the low literacy population is a strategy for obesity prevention.

Relationship between obesity and education outcomes in children and college students

Obese children are at risk for health problems later in adulthood, including diabetes, heart disease, and certain forms of cancer. The number of children overweight or obese is increasing globally, from 32 million in 1990 to 41 million in 2016 [3]. A child's upbringing, beginning from the mother's diet during pregnancy to food selection as toddler to feeding habits as child are critical steps in determining the risk of obesity in adulthood. Global urbanization and the use of digital methods of ordering and consuming foods means less opportunity for physical activities [13].

With rising obesity rates, understanding the relationship between academic performance and obesity can shed light on the relationship between obesity and educational outcomes. A number of studies published found a significant association between childhood obesity and poor academic performance [14]. Obesity is a factor in poor performance in children in grades K-12, and is linked to the overconsumption of energy and excess body mass with greater decay of brain structure function and brain aging [15]. Among high school students, school connectedness (participation in sports, work, etc.) has been linked to better adolescent health behaviors and a less sedentary lifestyle [16]. Studies linking obesity with academic performance in university students were examined among individuals between 19 and 30 years. In comparison to students not expecting to graduate from college, students fully expecting to graduate from college had 34% lower odds of being in the persistently overweight class (adjusted odds ratio = 0.66, 95% confidence interval = 0.54, 0.81), controlling for academic performance and socioeconomic status [16]. The diminished expectations for the future may undermine the adoption of positive health behaviors and those who expect to complete college educations are invested in healthier lifestyles and activities [17]. In university students, gender differences did not play a role in academic performance [18], but final grades did negatively correlate with BMI ($P=.001$) [18]. Individual students with BMIs >30 categorized as obese and BMI between 25 and 29 categorized as overweight did not perform well in school and were more likely to have a lower final grade than those students with BMIs in the normal or underweight categories [18].

Conclusion

Educational attainment may improve health outcomes depending on a country's development. Certain educational interventions can also be implemented to achieve weight loss. More governmental policies can be utilized to raise awareness of the impact of diet and exercise on weight loss.

Childhood obesity is also an area of concern, especially with the rise in obesity among school children. Special attention to dietary choices can impact future weight gain in adulthood. Children that are well connected to school activities such as sports or school clubs tend to have less likelihood of obesity. Such activity and engagement in school can raise their aspiration to enter and do well in college.

There is a gap in knowledge on the isolated effects of education separate from socioeconomic measures, and further studies are needed to elucidate such relations. Nevertheless, prospective studies are under way to directly measure the effects of lifestyle education on weight loss, which can support policy changes to support education in communities.

References

[1] Cohen AK, et al. Educational attainment and obesity: a systematic review. Obes Rev 2013;14 (12):989–1005. https://doi.org/10.1111/obr.12062.

[2] Roser M, Ortiz-Ospina E. Global education, Our World in Data; 2016 Aug. http://ourworldindata.org/global-education. [Accessed 13 February 2020].

[3] Kitagawa EM, Hauser PM. Differential mortality in the United States. Cambridge, MA: Harvard University Press; 1973.

[4] Adler NE, Rehkopf DH. U.S. disparities in health: descriptions, causes, and mechanisms. Annu Rev Public Health 2008;29:235–52.

[5] Chandola T, Clarke P, Morris J, Blane D. Pathways between education and health: a causal modeling approach. J R Stat Soc A Stat 2006;169(2):337–59.

[6] McLaren L. Socioeconomic status and obesity. Epidemiol Rev 2007;29:29–48.

[7] Miech R, Hauser R. Socioeconomic status and health at midlife: a comparison of educational attainment with occupation-based indicators. Ann Epidemiol 2001;11(2):75–84. PubMed: 11164123.

[8] Danzinger S, Gottschalk P, editors. Uneven tides: rising inequality in America. New York: Russell Sage; 1993.

[9] Sobal J, Stunkard AJ. Socioeconomic status and obesity: a review of the literature. Psychol Bull 1989;105:260–75.

[10] Hu EY, Ramachandran S, Bhattacharya K, Nunna S. Obesity among high school students in the United States: risk factors and their population attributable fraction, Prev Chronic Dis 2018;15:180122. https://doi.org/10.5888/pcd15.180122.

[11] Ostovan MA, Zibaeenezhad MJ, Keshmiri H, Shekarforoush S. The impact of education on weight loss in overweight and obese adults. Int Cardiovasc Res J 2013;7(3):79–82.

[12] Veghari G, et al. Influence of education in the prevalence of obesity in Iranian northern adults. J Cardiovasc Dis Res 2013;4(1):30–3. https://doi.org/10.1016/j.jcdr.2013.02.002.

[13] WHO. Facts and figures on childhood obesity. Updated: 2019 Sep. https://www.who.int/end-childhood-obesity/facts/en/. [Accessed 11 March 2020].

[14] ECD. The heavy burden of obesity: the economics of prevention. OECD Health Policy Studies. Paris: OECD Publishing; 2019. https://doi.org/10.1787/67450d67-en.

[15] Burkhalter TM, Hillman CH. A narrative review of physical activity, nutrition, and obesity to cognition and scholastic performance across the human lifespan. Adv Nutr 2011 Mar;2 (2):201S–206S. https://doi.org/10.3945/an.111.000331.

[16] Clarke PJ, O'Malley PM, Schulenberg JE, Lee H, Colabianchi N, Johnston LD. College expectations in high school mitigate weight gain over early adulthood: findings from a national study of American youth. Obesity 2013;21:1321–7. https://doi.org/10.1002/oby.20176.

[17] Jessor R, Donovan JE, Costa F. Personality, perceived life chances, and adolescent behavior. In: Hurrelmann K, Hamilton SF, editors. Social problems and social contexts in adolescence: perspectives across boundaries. Hawthorne, NY: Aldine de Gruyter; 1996. p. 219–33.

[18] Anderson AS, Good DJ. Increased body weight affects academic performance in university students. Prev Med Rep 2017;5:220–3. https://doi.org/10.1016/j.pmedr.2016.12.020.

Chapter 13

Refined food addiction and its relation to obesity

Lindsey G. Kahan, B.S. and Raman Mehrzad, M.D., M.H.L., M.B.A.
Department of Plastic and Reconstructive Surgery, Rhode Island Hospital, The Warren Alpert Medical School of Brown University, Providence, RI, United States

Introduction

With advances in manufacturing and global trade, mass-produced refined foods have globally increased in prevalence [1]. Additionally, our understanding of neurobiological models of addiction has improved due to more advanced computation and neuroimaging technology [2]. The analysis of the neurobiological and clinical frameworks for the consumption of refined foods has led to the exploration of addiction to refined foods and its association with the rise in global obesity.

Defining refined food

Refined food includes white bread, sugar, and sweetened beverages. Grains undergo a milling process to increase the surface area and glycemic index. By manufacturing whole grains into white flour, the caloric density increases by more than 10%, the fiber reduces by 80%, and the protein reduces by almost 30% [3]. Compared to their whole grain counterparts, refined carbohydrates are nearly pure starch with fewer nutrients.

In addition to refined carbohydrates, the processing of other food products has become more standardized throughout the global food industry. The UN General Assembly has defined ultraprocessed foods to refer to manufactured items that "contain little or no whole foods, are ready to consume or heat up, and are fatty, salty, or sugary and depleted in dietary fiber, protein, various micronutrients, and other bioactive compounds" [4]. The UN established NOVA, a food classification system based on the processing technique, that separates food items into four categories:

(1) unprocessed or minimally processed foods (e.g., seeds, fruits, leaves, animal muscle, milk).

Obesity. https://doi.org/10.1016/B978-0-12-818839-2.00013-2

(2) processed culinary ingredients (e.g., oils, butter, sugar, salt).
(3) processed foods including the addition of foods from Group 2 into Group 1 (e.g., bottled vegetables, canned fish, fruits in syrup, cheeses).
(4) ultraprocessed foods, which are formulations of mostly or entirely new substances (e.g., soft drinks, packaged snacks, reconstituted meat products, additives) [4].

Ultraprocessed food ingredients lack dietary fiber and water, thus increasing the energy density. They also generally carry higher glycemic indices, which has been correlated to lower satiety potential [5].

A changing global food climate

Rapid global urbanization has been accompanied by a change in diet of those in cities, showing trends of higher consumption of milled and processed grains, sugar, and processed foods [6]. Globally, low- and medium-income countries have adopted the "Western diet," which includes refined carbohydrates, added sugars, fats, and animal-sourced foods [7]. For example, in middle-income countries such as Brazil, Croatia, Slovakia, Hungary, Lithuania, and Latvia, ultraprocessed foods comprised a range of 18–33% of household food purchases [8, 9]. The availability of ultraprocessed food and obesity were positively associated (Fig. 1) [9]. As this transition has occurred, a phenomenon of the "dual burden" has emerged—underweight, stunting, and micronutrient deficiencies paralleling increasing rates of obesity [7].

Refined carbohydrates, and in particular corn syrup sweeteners, have significantly increased in prevalence in the United States [10]. From 1970 to 1997, there were dramatic increases in refined product consumption, including a 42% increase in corn and wheat flour, a 1240% increase in high fructose corn syrup, a 218% increase in carbonated soft drinks, and a 207% increase in frozen potatoes [11].

In the United States, ultraprocessed food products comprise 57.9% of the food supply and are responsible for nearly 90% of all added sugars [12]. About a quarter of US working adults access food at their workplace, which systemically has been shown to include foods that perform poorly on dietary quality scales. Workplace foods were found to be high in empty calories, sodium, and refined grains [13].

The prevalence of refined foods has increased due to the profitability of processed foods, which stems from their low production cost, long shelf-life, and high retail value [1]. Foods with lower nutritional value are more widely available and cheaper than those with higher nutritional value [14]. Globally, increases in highly processed foods, refined foods, and sugar-sweetened beverage consumption parallel increases in obesity and metabolic syndrome [15–19]. The consumption of ultraprocessed foods has been associated with an increased

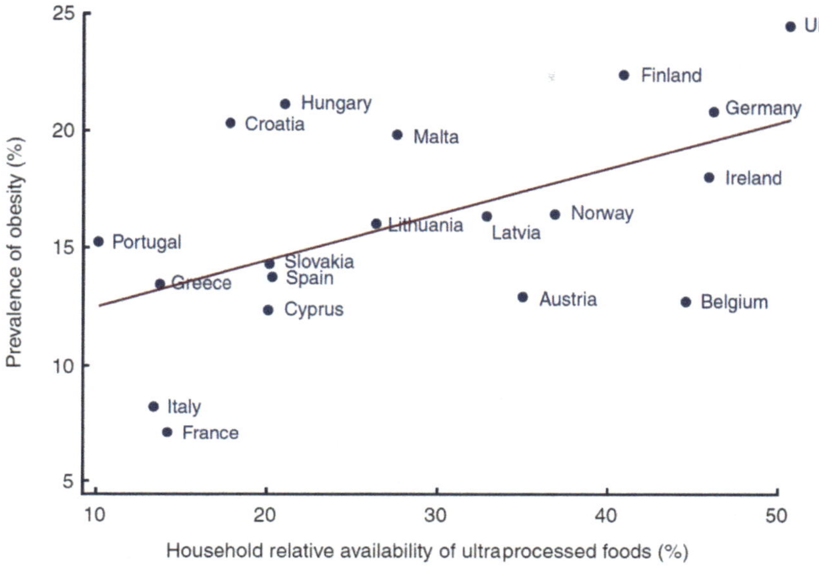

FIG. 1 Regression of the prevalence of obesity among adults vs. household availability of ultra-processed foods (percentage of total energy) in 19 European countries (1991–2008). *(Reproduced with permission from Monteiro CA, Moubarac J-C, Levy RB, Canella DS, da Costa Louzada ML, Cannon G, Household availability of ultra-processed foods and obesity in nineteen European countries. Public Health Nutr 2018 Jan;21(1):18–26. https://doi.org/10.1017/S1368980017001379 (web archive link).)*

risk of obesity, yet strong conclusions regarding the relationship cannot be made without more prospective studies [20]. While the driving factors for this parallel finding are likely multifactorial, the shift in global diet provides a framework for studying the association of refined foods to increasing global obesity rates.

Clinical classification of addiction

The term "addiction" has a variety of complex definitions, and has been classically applied to disorders of drugs and alcohol use [21]. The standard clinical method utilizes the Diagnostic and Statistical Manual of Mental Disorders, Fifth Edition (DSM-5), which uses 11 clinical biopsychosocial criteria to define substance use disorder. The criteria include hazardous use, social/interpersonal problems related to use, neglected major roles to use, withdrawal, tolerance, used larger amounts/longer, repeated attempts to quit/control use, much time spent using, physical/psychological problems related to use, activities given up to use, and craving [22]. In order to qualify for substance use disorder, more than two of the 11 listed criteria need to be present within a 12-month period.

TABLE 1 Diagnosis of substance use abuse, dependence, and disorders based on the DSM-4 and DSM-5.

	DSM-4	DSM-5
Hazardous use	Abuse ≥1	Substance use disorders Mild: 2–3; moderate: 4–5; severe: 6+
Social/interpersonal problems related to use		
Neglected major roles due to due		
Legal problems (replaced with craving in DSM-5)		
Withdrawal	Dependence ≥3	
Tolerance		
Increase in use		
Repeated attempts to quit/control use		
Much time spent using		
Physical/psychological problems related to use		
Activities given up due to use		

Criteria must be present within a 12-month period.
Adapted from Hasin DS, et al. DSM-5 criteria for substance use disorders: recommendations and rationale. Am J Psychiatry 2013 Aug;170(8):834–851. https://doi.org/10.1176/appi.ajp.2013.12060782.

From DSM 4 to 5, these criteria changed to incorporate abuse and dependence within one overarching substance use disorder diagnosis (Table 1) [23].

In addition to substance addictions, more research has elucidated behavioral addictions, or the dependence on a behavior or feeling brought on by an action. Behavioral and substance addictions have been shown to carry strong similarities in terms of both clinical actions and neurobiological mechanisms [21, 24, 25], leading to the new DSM-5 category of nonsubstance-related disorders. This category remains controversial in the literature, with several groups arguing for the incorporation of behaviors such as Internet gaming, shopping, sexual behaviors, and food addiction, and others suggesting a divergence between behavior and substance disorders. Currently, the DSM-5 only includes a gambling disorder, as other behavioral addictions such as food addiction were considered but were determined to be without sufficient evidence when the DSM-5 was introduced in 2013 [21, 24, 26, 27].

Food addiction: A potential link

While overeating may occur in a significant number of people, it has been shown that some individuals develop an addictive or obsessive relationship with food [28, 29]. As rates in refined sugar and obesity rise, our understanding of how these products affects the brain has also been analyzed. Animal studies have sought to understand the brain's response to food, glucose, and overeating for decades [30–33], and connections have developed in the literature between addiction and food.

The clinical appreciation for food addiction has also been studied to a greater degree in recent years, with the development of the Yale Food Addiction Scale (YFAS). The substance dependence criteria of DSM-4 was applied to eating behavior to standardize the diagnosis of food addition, and this is the only validated tool to assess food addiction (Table 2) [34, 35]. It has been applied to individuals to better understand the relationship between food addiction, obesity, and dietary patterns.

TABLE 2 Sample questions from the Yale Food Addiction Scale.

In the past 12 months:	Frequency
I find that when I start eating foods, I end up eating more than planned	Never Once a month 2–4 times a month 2–3 times a week 4 or more times per week or daily
Not eating certain types of food or cutting down on certain types of food is something I worry about	
I spend a lot of time feeling sluggish or lethargic from overeating	
I eat to the point where I feel physically ill	
There have been times when I avoided professional or social situations because I was not able to consume certain foods there	
My behavior with respect to food and eating causes significant distress	
I experience significant problems in my ability to function effectively because of food and eating	
There have been times when I consumed certain foods so often or in such large quantities that I spent time dealing with negative feelings from overeating instead of working, spending time with family/friends, or engaging in other important activities I enjoy	

Frequency reported for each question.
Adapted from Gearhardt AN, Corbin WR, Brownell KD. Preliminary validation of the Yale food addiction scale. Appetite 2009 Apr;52(2):430–436. https://doi.org/10.1016/j.appet.2008.12.003.

Neurobiology of addiction

With the increased understanding of neurobiological mechanisms of addiction, both the neurocircuitry and the molecular biology have been more completely worked out [36]. It has been well studied that reward processing and behavior involve the dopaminergic system, and that drugs with addictive potential increase the extracellular concentration of dopamine in the striatum and mesolimbic regions; these regions are thought to be the driving system of the positive reinforcing effects of drugs of abuse [36–38].

Ultimately, three stages have been identified within addictive patterns, each utilizing different neurocircuitry. The binge/intoxication phase, responsible for the acute reinforcement effects of a drug or behavior, most likely involves the nucleus accumbens-amygdala rewards system, dopaminergic inputs from the ventral tegmental area, and opioid peptide inputs. The withdrawal stage involves decreased function of the reward system, and the preoccupation/anticipation stage involves the amygdala and nucleus accumbens [36].

Neurobiological framework for food addiction

There has been an extensive look into uncovering the neural connections between patterns of food consumption and addiction [2]. Through the study of neurotransmitters, opioid receptors, fMRI, and EEG, brain responses to food have been better appreciated.

Dopamine

Several studies have analyzed brain chemistry changes in animal models in response to food. In rats, the overconsumption of highly palatable food was shown to activate neuroadaptive responses in brain reward circuits and drive compulsive eating in a similar manner to previously established responses of addiction [39, p. 2]. Highly palatable food included bacon, sausage, cheesecake, pound cake, frosting, and chocolate, which are consistent with processed and ultraprocessed foods [40]. Specifically, striatal dopamine D2 receptors were downregulated in obese rats, with similar reports in humans addicted to drugs [39, p. 2].

Further evidence for the link between food and addictive responses involves the study of excessive food, which relates to the problem of overeating. Intermittent excessive glucose intake in rats, when given in addition to a normal diet, increased activation of the dopamine D1 and mu-opioid-1 receptors, and decreased the dopamine D2 receptors [30]. These studies determined that dopaminergic patterns of excessive food intake were consistent with substance use disorder findings [34].

Altered dopamine pathways have also been implicated in human studies of individuals who qualified for a diagnosis of food addiction per the YFAS [34].

One study found that an appetite suppressant that blocked dopamine was ineffective in those who met food addiction per the YFAS criteria, suggesting altered dopamine signaling strength extraneous to dopamine itself; this finding was consistent with substance use disorders [41].

Opioid expression

The role of opioid receptors has been extensively analyzed in the study of substance use disorders. In terms of food intake, opioid receptors have been shown to play a role in food reward in animal studies [41, 42]. Gamma-aminobutyric acid (GABA) receptor activity has also been linked to food addiction through rat studies. It has been shown that rats given a GABA agonist and daily sweetened shortening ate significantly more chow than rats not fed the shortening [42]. Moreover, the repeated excessive intake of sugar in rats followed by abrupt withdrawal was shown to create a state of anxiety and dopamine/acetylcholine imbalance similar to that of opioid withdrawal [31]. In humans, it's been shown that in those with obesity and moderate binge eating, a mu-opioid receptor antagonist reduced motivation for high-calorie foods such as chocolate [43].

Neuroimaging

Imaging has revolutionized the study of neurobiology. It has been shown that foods and drugs activate similar brain regions on fMRI, particularly in obese individuals [44–47]. These findings, while providing insight into the pertinent similarities between food and drug response, don't adequately link food to addiction. One study utilized the DSM-4 substance abuse criteria to investigate food addiction to bridge this gap. Results showed that both lean and obese individuals with higher food addiction scores differentially displayed a pattern of neural activation from those with lower food addiction scores. The activation of brain regions in those with higher food addiction scores correlated with areas responsible for the motivational value of stimuli, and have been linked to substance dependence and craving [48].

Electroencephalogram

The relationship between YFAS symptoms of food addiction and substance use disorders has been appreciated through electroencephalogram (EEG) studies. One study found that three or more food addiction symptoms on the YFAS correlated with EEG changes similar to people with addictive disorders [49]. Additionally, when the resting-state EEG brain activity was analyzed between adults with obesity with YFAS symptoms (high YFAS), adults with obesity without YFAS symptoms (low YFAS), and adults with alcohol use disorder, there were findings suggestive of similarities between the high YFAS and alcohol use disorder groups [50]. This brain activity was determined to be pathological due to its absence in both the lean control group and the low YFAS group. This led to the conclusion that there are neurobiological similarities between food addiction symptoms and alcohol dependence, and that these addictions share a common neurophysiological substrate aside from the cellular, genetic, and behavioral aspects [50].

Clinical correlation: DSM-5 criteria

Impaired control

It has been repeatedly shown that individuals who suffer from overweight or obesity have a markedly difficult time losing weight [51], and that limiting intake or types of foods often does not produce the desired results. Even individuals who undergo bariatric surgery as a means of weight loss struggle with control over diet in the face of life-threatening consequences [52]. This demonstrates a failure of control consistent with substance use disorders [53]. The YFAS is a helpful tool for studying impaired control in the clinical setting; one study found that the number of addictive-like eating symptoms was associated with more difficulty controlling eating and less weight loss [54]. Other studies have found higher YFAS scores to be associated with food cravings, increased appetite following a taste of participants' favorite palatable food, and resistance to food-intake suppression following pharmacological challenge with a dopamine agonist [55–57].

Other clinical aspects of addiction include tolerance, withdrawal, time spent in the activity, and time given up on other activities due to the addicted behavior/substance. While impaired control has compelling evidence to suggest food addiction, these other categories lack empirical evidence. It has been suggested that the neurobiological framework of food addiction needs further research in order to bridge the gap to the behavioral disorder of food addiction [58]. Specifically, human studies need to be conducted in the behavioral dependence categories of withdrawal, tolerance, time spent in excess food consumption, and how important activities are given up due to food consumption [58].

Refined food and addiction

Through the aforementioned data, it has been established in the literature that food can activate brain change patterns similar to those seen in substance use disorders. However, what is critical to elicit is whether refined foods cause this behavior more than unrefined foods, and the clinical significance of these changes on a global scale.

The refined food addiction hypothesis, proposed by Ifland et al. in 2009, proposes that the same mechanisms that drive loss of control over drug use are also utilized in the loss of control over certain foods [29]. Through observations from interactions with self-identified refined food addicts, Ifland et al. administered a survey adapted from the DSM-4 substance dependence criteria. They demonstrated responses consistent with themes of tolerance, withdrawal, consuming refined foods more than intended, failure in cutting back, time spent recovering from use, missing important activities due to eating, and eating in spite of consequences [29]. To date, these findings have not been studied in more empirical trials.

To further explore the relationship between food type and addiction, addictive-like eating behaviors have been stratified by the food's absorption rate into the bloodstream, the glycemic load, and processing. It has been hypothesized that processed foods may harbor abuse potential in a similar mechanism to the processing of a coca leaf—not addictive when raw, but when concentrated into a rapid delivery system such as cocaine, it becomes highly addictive. Processed foods, with higher fat and glycemic load, had a greater association with addictive-like eating behaviors [59]. This hypothesis has yet to be adequately studied.

It has also been postulated that rather than a single macronutrient holding responsibility for addictive properties, an unnatural combination of macronutrients in palatable high-calorie foods may alter brain circuitry and create maladaptive responses [53]. One study showed that blended food containing a high amount of both fat and carbohydrates had a greater impact on reward centers in the brain than single-nutrient foods [60]. While the hypothesis that refined food has addictive properties that lead to obesity requires further quantitative validation, there exists current literature to support this theory.

Food addiction and obesity

It is important to separate the entities of food addiction and obesity. The YFAS is currently the only developed tool to assess food addiction [34], and several studies have utilized this tool to assess the relationship between addiction and obesity.

When a group of patients with obesity undergoing conservative weight loss treatment were studied, it was found that 32% of participants fit food addiction criteria per the YFAS [61]. Other estimates of food addiction have been reported as well. For example, when a general population in Newfoundland was studied, it was found that the prevalence of food addiction per the YFAS criteria was 5.4% [28]. When stratified by BMI, food addiction had a prevalence of 1.6% in under/normal weight and 7.7% in overweight/obese. Furthermore, obesity-related measurements such as BMI, weight, and various body measurements were found to have strong positive correlations with YFAS symptoms (Table 3) [28]. When controlling for age, sex, smoking, medication use, and physical activity, the Spearman partial correlation coefficients, a measure of nonparametric rank correlation between two variables, found a statistically significant correlation between food addiction and BMI and other obesity

TABLE 3 Correlation r between food addiction symptoms as measured by YFAS and obesity measurements.

		BMI (kg/m²)	Weight (kg)	% body fat
Entire cohort	*r*	0.36*	0.35*	0.31*
Nonfood addiction	*r*	0.32*	0.30*	0.27*

*$P < .001$.
Adapted from Pedram P, et al. Food addiction: its prevalence and significant association with obesity in the general population. PLoS One 2013;8(9):e74832. https://doi.org/10.1371/journal.pone.0074832.

measures (Table 3) [28]. Other studies have shown that YFAS food addiction is associated with higher current and lifetime BMI [62].

A systematic review that analyzed the prevalence of food addiction diagnosis found that within the food addiction literature, 24.9% of people with overweight/obesity qualified for a food addiction diagnosis, and 11.1% of healthy weight individuals qualified (Table 4) [34]. The fact that only a quarter of those with obesity had a food addiction limits the applicability of data that use obesity as a proxy for addiction. Other studies have argued against overeating as a mechanism for obesity by showing no correlation between YFAS scores and BMI [48] or by measuring brain patterns unsupportive of a food addiction model of overeating [43]. It has also been suggested that the addiction model

TABLE 4 Metaanalysis results of food addiction prevalence by weight.

Population group (*n* = No. of studies)	Weighted mean prevalence of food addiction diagnosis (%)	95% confidence interval (%)	Range of prevalence (%)
Total (*n* = 20)	19.9	16.3–24.0	5.4–56.8
Healthy weight (*n* = 5)	11.1	6.3–18.9	1.6–24.0
Overweight/obese (*n* = 13)	24.9	14.2–40.1	7.7–56.8

Adapted from Pursey K, Stanwell P, Gearhardt A, Collins C, Burrows T. The prevalence of food addiction as assessed by the Yale food addiction scale: a systematic review. Nutrients 2014 Oct;6(10):4552–4590. https://doi.org/10.3390/nu6104552.

of food, while holding convincing evidence in animal studies, has not translated to humans. The majority of overweight individuals have not shown behavioral or neurobiological phenomena consistent with addiction [63]. Further research using the YFAS and obesity needs to be conducted to fully elucidate the relationship between food types, addiction, and obesity [64]. Additionally, the Palatable Motives Eating Scale (PEMS), a validated scale for identifying motivations for palatable foods [65], should be utilized in conjunction with YFAS to build a comprehensive understanding of food addiction [64].

Food addiction and obesity in children

While most of the populations studied with the YFAS tool have been white adults, the criteria have also been applied to other populations to observe epidemiological differences among groups. One particularly important group to study is children, given that a child with obesity is more likely to have obesity as an adult. Furthermore, by validating the YFAS for children, it would enable the longitudinal study of food addiction [66].

In a group of African American adolescents with obesity, it was found that about 10% of participants met YFAS for children (YFAS-C) food addiction criteria [67]. Higher YFAS-C scores were significantly associated with greater consumption of all food characteristics such as sugar and carbohydrates; scores were most strongly associated with an increase in trans fats, which are common in refined foods. Those meeting YFAS-C diagnosis also reported significantly more objective binge episodes [67].

Other studies have shown food addiction prevalence rates of 8.9% in a Hungarian group of children [68], 4.5% in a group of Russian adolescents [69], and 22.7% in a group of parentally reported online survey participants [70]. Children's food addiction symptoms were found to be associated with parental food addiction symptoms, parental restrictive feeding practices (i.e., limiting access to unhealthy food), and parental pressure to eat feeding practices [70].

Food addiction and mental health

The relationship between mental health, food addiction, and obesity is important to fully elucidate. It has been shown that there is an increased rate of food addiction in adolescents with moderate-to-severe depression, highlighting the link between mental health and food addiction [69]. Moreover, in adolescent psychiatric inpatients, it was found that not only did these patients have higher rates of food addiction than seen in community samples of children, but food addiction was associated with eating disorders and disinhibition. However, no relationship was shown between food addiction and psychiatric disorders other than eating disorders [71].

A metaanalysis on 53 articles studying food addiction associations with mental health symptoms revealed that there are positive, moderate associations between food addiction and binge eating, depression, and anxiety. Fewer studies reported on associations between food addiction, PTSD, and emotional eating [72].

Food addiction and eating disorders

It has previously been observed that the prevalence of eating disorders is higher among people with overweight and obesity compared to people with BMIs within the normal range. Additionally, the prevalence of eating disorders has been increasing in recent decades, as has obesity with comorbid binge eating, potentially highlighting the need to study integrated approaches to these conditions [62, 73].

Several eating disorders have been studied in association with food addiction. For example, bulimia has been found to have the highest prevalence of food addiction compared to those with anorexia, binge eating disorder, and obesity with or without binge eating disorder [74]. There exists significant overlap between those with diagnostic YFAS criteria and those with binge eating disorder, as diagnosed by the Binge Eating Scale (BES) [75]. 72% of participants with food addiction had either moderate or severe binging, comparing to 9.9% of participants without food addiction. An overall correlation between food addiction and BES scores was found to be $r = 0.76$, demonstrating a significant overlap [75].

Other studies have also demonstrated clinically significant food addiction and have reported ranges of food addiction between 41.5% and 57% within groups of patients with binge eating disorder and obesity. Moreover, these patients had significantly higher levels of depression and emotion dysregulation as well as lower self-esteem [76, 77]. In a systematic review of the food addiction literature, it was reported that of those diagnosed with an eating disorder, the prevalence of food addiction was 57.6% compared to 16.2% without a clinically diagnosed eating disorder [34].

Summary

Hyperpalatable food, including ultraprocessed and refined foods, has been shown to stimulate similar neurobiological mechanisms that underlie drug and alcohol addiction. Which foods exhibit the most addictive potential, while preliminarily studied, still lacks a clear answer. Additionally, no single source of addictive substance has been identified and the appropriateness of the application of the neurobiological components to clinical practice remains unclear. The development of the YFAS and its potential linkage to refined foods could further elucidate patterns of overeating and obesity.

References

[1] Stuckler D, McKee M, Ebrahim S, Basu S. Manufacturing epidemics: the role of global producers in increased consumption of unhealthy commodities including processed foods, alcohol, and tobacco. PLoS Med 2012 Jun;9(6):e1001235. https://doi.org/10.1371/journal.pmed.1001235.

[2] Volkow ND, Wang G-J, Tomasi D, Baler RD. Obesity and addiction: neurobiological overlaps: overlaps between drug and food addiction. Obes Rev 2013 Jan;14(1):2–18. https://doi.org/10.1111/j.1467-789X.2012.01031.x.

[3] Durtschi A. Nutritional content of whole grains versus their refined flours. Walton Feed Company. USDA Economic Research Service; 2001 Feb.

[4] Monteiro CA, Cannon G, Moubarac J-C, Levy RB, Louzada MLC, Jaime PC. The UN decade of nutrition, the NOVA food classification and the trouble with ultra-processing. Public Health Nutr 2018 Jan;21(1):5–17. https://doi.org/10.1017/S1368980017000234.

[5] Fardet A. Minimally processed foods are more satiating and less hyperglycemic than ultra-processed foods: a preliminary study with 98 ready-to-eat foods. Food Funct 2016;7(5):2338–46. https://doi.org/10.1039/C6FO00107F.

[6] Popkin BM. The nutrition transition and its health implications in lower-income countries. Public Health Nutr 1998 Mar;1(1):5–21. https://doi.org/10.1079/PHN19980004.

[7] Popkin BM, Adair LS, Ng SW. Global nutrition transition and the pandemic of obesity in developing countries. Nutr Rev 2012 Jan;70(1):3–21. https://doi.org/10.1111/j.1753-4887.2011.00456.x.

[8] da Costa Louzada ML, et al. Ultra-processed foods and the nutritional dietary profile in Brazil. Rev Saude Publica 2015;49:38. https://doi.org/10.1590/S0034-8910.2015049006132.

[9] Monteiro CA, Moubarac J-C, Levy RB, Canella DS, da Costa Louzada ML, Cannon G. Household availability of ultra-processed foods and obesity in nineteen European countries. Public Health Nutr 2018 Jan;21(1):18–26. https://doi.org/10.1017/S1368980017001379.

[10] Gross LS, Li L, Ford ES, Liu S. Increased consumption of refined carbohydrates and the epidemic of type 2 diabetes in the United States: an ecologic assessment. Am J Clin Nutr 2004 May;79(5):774–9. https://doi.org/10.1093/ajcn/79.5.774.

[11] Putnam J, Allshouse J. Food consumption, prices and expenditures. United States Department of Agriculture; 1999. No. 965.

[12] Martínez Steele E, Baraldi LG, da Costa Louzada ML, Moubarac J-C, Mozaffarian D, Monteiro CA. Ultra-processed foods and added sugars in the US diet: evidence from a nationally representative cross-sectional study. BMJ Open 2016 Jan;6(3):e009892. https://doi.org/10.1136/bmjopen-2015-009892.

[13] Onufrak SJ, Zaganjor H, Pan L, Lee-Kwan SH, Park S, Harris DM. Foods and beverages obtained at worksites in the United States. J Acad Nutr Diet 2019 Jun;119(6):999–1008. https://doi.org/10.1016/j.jand.2018.11.011.

[14] Jetter KM, Cassady DL. The availability and cost of healthier food alternatives. Am J Prev Med 2006 Jan;30(1):38–44. https://doi.org/10.1016/j.amepre.2005.08.039.

[15] Brownell KD, Frieden TR. Ounces of prevention–the public policy case for taxes on sugared beverages. N Engl J Med 2009 Apr;360(18):1805–8. https://doi.org/10.1056/NEJMp0902392.

[16] DeBres K. Burgers for Britain: a cultural geography of McDonald's UK. J Cult Geogr 2005 Mar;22(2):115–39. https://doi.org/10.1080/08873630509478241.

[17] Ludwig DS, Peterson KE, Gortmaker SL. Relation between consumption of sugar-sweetened drinks and childhood obesity: a prospective, observational analysis. Lancet 2001 Feb;357(9255):505–8. https://doi.org/10.1016/S0140-6736(00)04041-1.

[18] Vartiainen E, et al. Thirty-five-year trends in cardiovascular risk factors in Finland. Int J Epidemiol 2010 Apr;39(2):504–18. https://doi.org/10.1093/ije/dyp330.

[19] Bray GA, Nielsen SJ, Popkin BM. Consumption of high-fructose corn syrup in beverages may play a role in the epidemic of obesity. Am J Clin Nutr 2004 Apr;79(4):537–43. https://doi.org/10.1093/ajcn/79.4.537.

[20] Poti JM, Braga B, Qin B. Ultra-processed food intake and obesity: what really matters for health—processing or nutrient content? Curr Obes Rep 2017 Dec;6(4):420–31. https://doi.org/10.1007/s13679-017-0285-4.

[21] Gordon E, Ariel-Donges A, Bauman V, Merlo L. What is the evidence for 'food addiction?' A systematic review. Nutrients 2018 Apr;10(4):477. https://doi.org/10.3390/nu10040477.

[22] American Psychiatric Association and American Psychiatric Association, editor. Diagnostic and statistical manual of mental disorders: DSM-5. 5th ed. Washington, DC: American Psychiatric Association; 2013. eds.

[23] Hasin DS, et al. DSM-5 criteria for substance use disorders: recommendations and rationale. Am J Psychiatry 2013 Aug;170(8):834–51. https://doi.org/10.1176/appi.ajp.2013.12060782.

[24] Konkolÿ Thege B, Woodin EM, Hodgins DC, Williams RJ. Natural course of behavioral addictions: a 5-year longitudinal study. BMC Psychiatry 2015 Dec;15(1):4. https://doi.org/10.1186/s12888-015-0383-3.

[25] Olsen CM. Natural rewards, neuroplasticity, and non-drug addictions. Neuropharmacology 2011 Dec;61(7):1109–22. https://doi.org/10.1016/j.neuropharm.2011.03.010.

[26] Moreno C, Tandon R. Should overeating and obesity be classified as an addictive disorder in DSM-5? Curr Pharm Des 2011 Apr;17(12):1128–31. https://doi.org/10.2174/138161211795656701.

[27] Potenza MN. Non-substance addictive behaviors in the context of DSM-5. Addict Behav 2014 Jan;39(1):1–2. https://doi.org/10.1016/j.addbeh.2013.09.004.

[28] Pedram P, et al. Food addiction: its prevalence and significant association with obesity in the general population. PLoS One 2013 Sep;8(9):e74832. https://doi.org/10.1371/journal.pone.0074832.

[29] Ifland JR, et al. Refined food addiction: a classic substance use disorder. Med Hypotheses 2009 May;72(5):518–26. https://doi.org/10.1016/j.mehy.2008.11.035.

[30] Colantuoni C, et al. Excessive sugar intake alters binding to dopamine and mu-opioid receptors in the brain. Neuroreport 2001 Nov;12(16):3549–52. https://doi.org/10.1097/00001756-200111160-00035.

[31] Colantuoni C, et al. Evidence that intermittent, excessive sugar intake causes endogenous opioid dependence. Obes Res 2002 Jun;10(6):478–88. https://doi.org/10.1038/oby.2002.66.

[32] Specker SM, Lac ST, Carroll ME. Food deprivation history and cocaine self-administration: an animal model of binge eating. Pharmacol Biochem Behav 1994 Aug;48(4):1025–9. https://doi.org/10.1016/0091-3057(94)90215-1.

[33] Hagan MM, Moss DE. An animal model of bulimia nervosa: opioid sensitivity to fasting episodes. Pharmacol Biochem Behav 1991 Jun;39(2):421–2. https://doi.org/10.1016/0091-3057(91)90201-C.

[34] Pursey K, Stanwell P, Gearhardt A, Collins C, Burrows T. The prevalence of food addiction as assessed by the Yale food addiction scale: a systematic review. Nutrients 2014 Oct;6(10):4552–90. https://doi.org/10.3390/nu6104552.

[35] Gearhardt AN, Corbin WR, Brownell KD. Preliminary validation of the Yale food addiction scale. Appetite 2009 Apr;52(2):430–6. https://doi.org/10.1016/j.appet.2008.12.003.

[36] Koob GF, Simon EJ. The neurobiology of addiction: where we have been and where we are going. J Drug Issues 2009 Jan;39(1):115–32. https://doi.org/10.1177/002204260903900110.

[37] Di Chiara G. Nucleus accumbens shell and core dopamine: differential role in behavior and addiction. Behav Brain Res 2002 Dec;137(1–2):75–114. https://doi.org/10.1016/S0166-4328(02)00286-3.

[38] Koob GF. Drugs of abuse: anatomy, pharmacology and function of reward pathways. Trends Pharmacol Sci 1992 May;13(5):177–84. https://doi.org/10.1016/0165-6147(92)90060-j.

[39] Johnson PM, Kenny PJ. Dopamine D2 receptors in addiction-like reward dysfunction and compulsive eating in obese rats. Nat Neurosci 2010 May;13(5):635–41. https://doi.org/10.1038/nn.2519.

[40] Epstein DH, Shaham Y. Cheesecake-eating rats and the question of food addiction. Nat Neurosci 2010 May;13(5):529–31. https://doi.org/10.1038/nn0510-529.

[41] Le Merrer J, Stephens DN. Food-induced behavioral sensitization, its cross-sensitization to cocaine and morphine, pharmacological blockade, and effect on food intake. J Neurosci 2006 Jul;26(27):7163–71. https://doi.org/10.1523/JNEUROSCI.5345-05.2006.

[42] Newman S, Pascal L, Sadeghian K, Baldo BA. Sweetened-fat intake sensitizes gamma-aminobutyric acid—mediated feeding responses elicited from the nucleus Accumbens Shell. Biol Psychiatry 2013 May;73(9):843–50. https://doi.org/10.1016/j.biopsych.2012.11.027.

[43] Cambridge VC, et al. Neural and behavioral effects of a novel mu opioid receptor antagonist in binge-eating obese people. Biol Psychiatry 2013 May;73(9):887–94. https://doi.org/10.1016/j.biopsych.2012.10.022.

[44] Stice E, Spoor S, Ng J, Zald DH. Relation of obesity to consummatory and anticipatory food reward. Physiol Behav 2009 Jul;97(5):551–60. https://doi.org/10.1016/j.physbeh.2009.03.020.

[45] Stoeckel LE, Weller RE, Cook EW, Twieg DB, Knowlton RC, Cox JE. Widespread reward-system activation in obese women in response to pictures of high-calorie foods. Neuroimage 2008 Jun;41(2):636–47. https://doi.org/10.1016/j.neuroimage.2008.02.031.

[46] Rothemund Y, et al. Differential activation of the dorsal striatum by high-calorie visual food stimuli in obese individuals. Neuroimage 2007 Aug;37(2):410–21. https://doi.org/10.1016/j.neuroimage.2007.05.008.

[47] Volkow ND, et al. Cocaine cues and dopamine in dorsal striatum: mechanism of craving in cocaine addiction. J Neurosci 2006 Jun;26(24):6583–8. https://doi.org/10.1523/JNEUROSCI.1544-06.2006.

[48] Gearhardt AN. Neural correlates of food addiction. Arch Gen Psychiatry 2011 Aug;68(8):808. https://doi.org/10.1001/archgenpsychiatry.2011.32.

[49] Imperatori C, et al. Modification of EEG functional connectivity and EEG power spectra in overweight and obese patients with food addiction: an eLORETA study. Brain Imaging Behav 2015 Dec;9(4):703–16. https://doi.org/10.1007/s11682-014-9324-x.

[50] De Ridder D, et al. The brain, obesity and addiction: an EEG neuroimaging study. Sci Rep 2016 Dec;6(1):34122. https://doi.org/10.1038/srep34122.

[51] Puhl RM, Moss-Racusin CA, Schwartz MB, Brownell KD. Weight stigmatization and bias reduction: perspectives of overweight and obese adults. Health Educ Res 2007 Apr;23(2):347–58. https://doi.org/10.1093/her/cym052.

[52] Saunders R. Compulsive eating and gastric bypass surgery: what does hunger have to do with it? Obes Surg 2001 Dec;11(6):757–61. https://doi.org/10.1381/09608920160558731.

[53] Fletcher PC, Kenny PJ. Food addiction: a valid concept? Neuropsychopharmacology 2018 Dec;43(13):2506–13. https://doi.org/10.1038/s41386-018-0203-9.

[54] Burmeister JM, Hinman N, Koball A, Hoffmann DA, Carels RA. Food addiction in adults seeking weight loss treatment. Implications for psychosocial health and weight loss. Appetite 2013 Jan;60:103–10. https://doi.org/10.1016/j.appet.2012.09.013.

[55] Davis C, Curtis C, Levitan RD, Carter JC, Kaplan AS, Kennedy JL. Evidence that 'food addiction' is a valid phenotype of obesity. Appetite 2011 Dec;57(3):711–7. https://doi.org/10.1016/j.appet.2011.08.017.

[56] Davis C, Levitan RD, Kaplan AS, Kennedy JL, Carter JC. Food cravings, appetite, and snack-food consumption in response to a psychomotor stimulant drug: the moderating effect of 'food-addiction'. Front Psychol 2014;5:403. https://doi.org/10.3389/fpsyg.2014.00403.

[57] Davis C, Loxton NJ, Levitan RD, Kaplan AS, Carter JC, Kennedy JL. 'Food addiction' and its association with a dopaminergic multilocus genetic profile. Physiol Behav 2013 Jun;118:63–9. https://doi.org/10.1016/j.physbeh.2013.05.014.

[58] Gearhardt AN, Corbin WR, Brownell KD. Food addiction: an examination of the diagnostic criteria for dependence. J Addict Med 2009 Mar;3(1):1–7. https://doi.org/10.1097/ADM.0b013e318193c993.

[59] Schulte EM, Avena NM, Gearhardt AN. Which foods may be addictive? The roles of processing, fat content, and glycemic load. PLoS One 2015 Feb;10(2):e0117959. https://doi.org/10.1371/journal.pone.0117959.

[60] DiFeliceantonio AG, et al. Supra-additive effects of combining fat and carbohydrate on food reward. Cell Metab 2018 Jul;28(1):33–44.e3. https://doi.org/10.1016/j.cmet.2018.05.018.

[61] Locatelli L, Pataky Z, Boulanouar L, Golay A. Food addiction in patients with obesity. J Obes Eat Disord 2019 Oct;5(2):3. https://doi.org/10.36648/2471-8203.5.2.100043.

[62] Gearhardt AN, Boswell RG, White MA. The association of 'food addiction' with disordered eating and body mass index. Eat Behav 2014 Aug;15(3):427–33. https://doi.org/10.1016/j.eatbeh.2014.05.001.

[63] Ziauddeen H, Farooqi IS, Fletcher PC. Obesity and the brain: how convincing is the addiction model? Nat Rev Neurosci 2012 Apr;13(4):279–86. https://doi.org/10.1038/nrn3212.

[64] Lerma-Cabrera JM, Carvajal F, Lopez-Legarrea P. Food addiction as a new piece of the obesity framework. Nutr J 2015 Dec;15(1):5. https://doi.org/10.1186/s12937-016-0124-6.

[65] Burgess EE, Turan B, Lokken KL, Morse A, Boggiano MM. Profiling motives behind hedonic eating. Preliminary validation of the palatable eating motives scale. Appetite 2014 Jan;72:66–72. https://doi.org/10.1016/j.appet.2013.09.016.

[66] Schiestl ET, Gearhardt AN. Preliminary validation of the Yale food addiction scale for children 2.0: a dimensional approach to scoring. Eur Eat Disord Rev 2018;26(6):605–17. https://doi.org/10.1002/erv.2648.

[67] Schulte EM, Jacques-Tiura AJ, Gearhardt AN, Naar S. Food addiction prevalence and concurrent validity in African American adolescents with obesity. Psychol Addict Behav 2018 Mar;32(2):187–96. https://doi.org/10.1037/adb0000325.

[68] Magyar ÉE, et al. Adaptation and validation of the Hungarian version of the Yale food addiction scale for children. J Behav Addict 2018 Mar;7(1):181–8. https://doi.org/10.1556/2006.7.2018.03.

[69] Borisenkov MF, Tserne TA, Bakutova LA. Food addiction in Russian adolescents: associations with age, sex, weight, and depression. Eur Eat Disord Rev 2018;26(6):671–6. https://doi.org/10.1002/erv.2644.

[70] Burrows T, Skinner J, Joyner M, Palmieri J, Vaughan K, Gearhardt A. Food addiction in children: associations with obesity, parental food addiction and feeding practices. Eat Behav 2017 Aug;26:114–20. https://doi.org/10.1016/j.eatbeh.2017.02.004.

[71] Albayrak Ö, et al. Eating-related psychopathology and food addiction in adolescent psychiatric inpatients. Eur Eat Disord Rev 2017;25(3):214–20. https://doi.org/10.1002/erv.2509.

[72] Burrows T, Kay-Lambkin F, Pursey K, Skinner J, Dayas C. Food addiction and associations with mental health symptoms: a systematic review with meta-analysis. J Hum Nutr Diet 2018;31(4):544–72. https://doi.org/10.1111/jhn.12532.

[73] da Luz FQ, Sainsbury A, Mannan H, Touyz S, Mitchison D, Hay P. Prevalence of obesity and comorbid eating disorder behaviors in South Australia from 1995 to 2015. Int J Obes (Lond) 2017 Jul;41(7):1148–53. https://doi.org/10.1038/ijo.2017.79.

[74] de Vries S-K, Meule A. Food addiction and bulimia nervosa: new data based on the Yale food addiction scale 2.0: food addiction and bulimia. Eur Eat Disord Rev 2016 Nov;24(6):518–22. https://doi.org/10.1002/erv.2470.

[75] Burrows T, Skinner J, McKenna R, Rollo M. Food addiction, binge eating disorder, and obesity: is there a relationship? Behav Sci 2017 Aug;7(4):54. https://doi.org/10.3390/bs7030054.

[76] Gearhardt AN, White MA, Masheb RM, Morgan PT, Crosby RD, Grilo CM. An examination of the food addiction construct in obese patients with binge eating disorder. Int J Eat Disord 2012 Jul;45(5):657–63. https://doi.org/10.1002/eat.20957.

[77] Gearhardt AN, White MA, Masheb RM, Grilo CM. An examination of food addiction in a racially diverse sample of obese patients with binge eating disorder in primary care settings. Compr Psychiatry 2013 Jul;54(5):500–5. https://doi.org/10.1016/j.comppsych.2012.12.009.

Chapter 14

Glycemic index

David Kim, M.D.
Department of Surgery, Rhode Island Hospital, Alpert Medical School of Brown University, Providence, RI, United States

Introduction

Despite local, national, and global public health efforts in addressing the obesity pandemic, the rates of obesity continue to rise with >40% of adults in most Western societies now being overweight or obese. In fact, since the early 1980s, the rate of individuals who are overweight or obese has approximately doubled [1]. As such, there has been considerable interest in better understanding the complex interplay of genetic, environmental, and socioeconomic factors that may be driving this alarming increase in the number of overweight and obese individuals.

Environmental factors such as food intake and highly processed carbohydrate foods can contribute to weight gain [2]. Given the implications on weight gain, overeating, and overall health, dietary carbohydrates, including the type and quantity, have been rigorously studied in the scientific community.

Definition

The glycemic index (GI) is one of several values used to measure how rapidly the body digests or breaks down carbohydrates [2]. More specifically, the GI value describes the effect of a carbohydrate-containing food on serum glucose following the consumption of that food.

The term was first introduced by Jenkins et al. in 1981 in a paper titled "Glycemic index of foods: a physiological basis for carbohydrate exchange." At the time, carbohydrate exchange lists designed by the American Diabetes Association and the American Dietetic Association were used to count carbohydrates and help with meal planning among diabetics, exchanging foods with similar amounts of carbohydrates. One of the primary principles in managing diabetics included tight glycemic control to reduce the long-term complications associated with the disease. Although the carbohydrate exchange lists were

Obesity. https://doi.org/10.1016/B978-0-12-818839-2.00014-4

helpful, they did not necessarily reflect the body's physiological blood glucose response following the consumption of commonly eaten foods [3].

Jenkins and his colleagues generated dose–response curves of 62 commonly eaten foods and sugars in healthy volunteers. Using these curves, they defined the GI value of a food as the incremental area under the 2h blood glucose response curve after consumption of a food containing 50g of available carbohydrates expressed as a percentage of the area after taking the same amount of carbohydrate as a reference food, such as white bread or pure glucose [3].

Interpretation of GI values

The GI of a particular food is a value that ranges from 0 to 100 with a low GI interpreted as 55 or less, a medium GI between 56 and 69, and a high GI as 70 or more (Tables 1 and 2).

Low-GI foods are digested and absorbed more slowly, causing a slower and steadier increase in blood glucose levels. High-GI foods are digested and absorbed more quickly, leading to a more rapid increase in blood glucose levels [4]. For example, vegetables, fruits, and legumes tend to have a low GI, whereas refined grain products and potatoes generally have a high GI (Fig. 1).

The GI value is affected by the carbohydrate type, fiber, protein, fat, and food form, among many other factors [5]. For example, the GI value of many fruits increases as they ripen with time [6]. The cooking time for pasta can also impact its final GI value, that is, a longer cooking time would increase the GI value. Additionally, the combination of high-GI and low-GI foods can lower the overall GI value, slowing down the rise in blood glucose levels. Finally, a person's individual characteristics such as age, metabolism, and overall health may impact the GI value [6].

In 1997, according to the World Health Organization and the Food and Agriculture Organization of the United Nations, an expert committee reviewed

TABLE 1 How to interpret glycemic index (GI) and glycemic load (GL).

Glycemic index	Glycemic load
The smaller the number, the less impact the food has on your blood sugar	The smaller the number, the less impact the food has on your blood sugar per serving size
55 or less = low	10 or less = low
56–69 = moderate	11–19 = moderate
70 or higher = high	20 or more = high

Foods that have a low GL almost always have a low GI. Foods with an intermediate or high GL range from a very low to very high GI.
From Rakel D. Glycemic index and glycemic load. Integrative medicine. Elsevier; 2018. p. 863–868.e1 [Chapter 87].

TABLE 2 Glycemic index of foods.

Low GI foods (55 or less)	Stone-ground whole wheat or pumpernickel bread, oatmeal (rolled or steel-cut), oat bran, muesli, pasta, converted rice, barley, bulgur, sweet potato, corn, yam, lima/butter beans, peas, legumes, lentils, most fruits, nonstarchy vegetables, and carrots
Medium GI (56 to 69)	Whole wheat, rye, pita bread, quick oats, brown, wild, or basmati rice, couscous
High GI (70 or more)	White bread or bagel, corn flakes, puffed rice, bran flakes, instant oatmeal, short grain white rice, rice pasta, macaroni and cheese from mix, Russet potato, pumpkin, pretzels, rice cakes, popcorn, saltine crackers, melons, and pineapple

From the American Diabetes Association: https://www.diabetes.org/glycemic-index-and-diabetes.

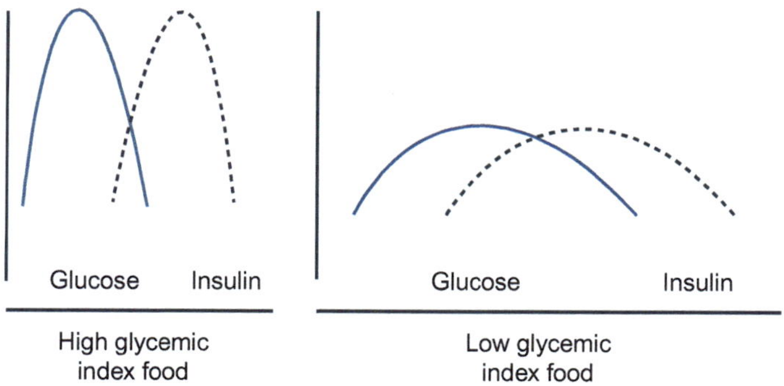

FIG. 1 The effect of high glycemic index food versus low glycemic food on glucose and insulin. *(From Rakel D. Glycemic index and glycemic load. Integrative medicine. Elsevier; 2018. p. 863–868.e1 [Chapter 87].)*

the existing literature and scientific evidence regarding the value of carbohydrates in nutrition and health. That committee recommended the use of GI values for classifying carbohydrate-rich foods. In addition, the committee recommended using GI values and food composition information to guide dietary planning [7].

Glycemic load

The concept of glycemic load (GL) was later introduced by Salmeron et al. at Harvard University in 1997 to account for the contribution of not only the type of carbohydrate (i.e., glycemic index) but additionally the amount of available carbohydrates per serving to the overall glycemic response [8]. The GL of a food is defined as the product of the GI value of the food and the amount of available carbohydrates in grams per serving of that food [9]. It is important to note that serving size is variable based on dietary and cultural factors [6]. Therefore, a food with a higher GL is expected to raise the serum glucose and insulin response per serving size to a greater extent than that of a food with a lower GL. A glycemic load value of 10 or less is considered low, 11–19 is considered medium, and 20 or more is considered high.

Appetite

Multiple published studies have demonstrated an association between GI and appetite. Compared to high-GI foods, low-GI foods have been associated with increased satiety, delayed return of hunger, and decreased ad lib food intake [5], all of which contribute to weight control.

Obesity and weight management

High-GI foods promote postprandial hyperglycemia and hyperinsulinemia, which lead to storage of nutrients in fat and weight gain [5], whereas low-GI foods may aid in weight control by promoting satiety as well as regulating postprandial insulin secretion and maintaining insulin sensitivity [1]. Additionally, high-GI foods are associated with hormonal responses that effectively stimulate hunger, leading to excessive weight gain. In a study conducted by Ludwig and colleagues in obese teenage boys, the group examined the effects of dietary GI on energy metabolism and voluntary food intake. They discovered that the rapid absorption of glucose following the consumption of high-GI meals induces a sequence of hormonal and metabolic changes that lead to overeating (Fig. 2) [10].

A diet focused on a lower GL and increased protein intake has been implicated in weight loss for those who are overweight or obese. According to a study conducted in the Chicago metropolitan area, Maki and colleagues found that overweight and obese adults on an ad lib reduced-glycemic-load diet demonstrated a statistically significant weight loss at 12 weeks, compared to those adhering to a traditional, low-fat portion-controlled diet [11].

Noninsulin-dependent diabetes mellitus

Noninsulin-dependent diabetes mellitus (NIDDM) is characterized by hyperglycemia; insulin resistance, which is a decrease in the effect of insulin on peripheral tissues; and relative insulin deficiency. Identifying potential dietary modifications to attenuate the risk of developing NIDDM has been an area of interest. Several studies, including a prospective study by Salmeron et al. from Harvard University, have shown that the consumption of high-GI carbohydrates and high GL are positively associated with a risk of NIDDM in both men and

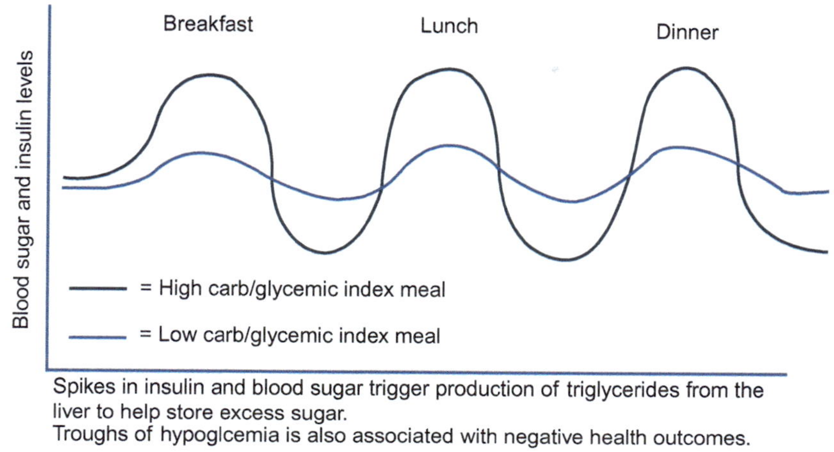

FIG. 2 Blood sugar and insulin levels. *(From Rakel D. Glycemic index and glycemic load. Integrative medicine. Elsevier; 2018. p. 863–868.e1 [Chapter 87].)*

women, whereas the intake of cereal fiber is inversely associated with a risk of NIDDM [8]. Additionally, the combination of a high GL and a low cereal fiber diet was associated with a higher risk of diabetes in the studied cohort [8].

Coronary heart disease

Diets with lower amounts of carbohydrates oftentimes contain higher amounts of fat and protein, which is associated with an adverse lipid profile. This shift in nutrient balance was once thought to be detrimental to a person's risk of developing coronary heart disease. A 2006 study published in the New England Journal of Medicine demonstrated that low-carbohydrate diets containing higher amounts of protein and fat are not associated with an increased risk of coronary heart disease [12]. Additionally, a prospective study conducted by the same group concluded that diets with a high GL independently increase the risk of coronary heart disease [13].

Oxidative stress and inflammation

Obesity is thought to instigate oxidative stress and inflammation, which have been linked to insulin resistance and cardiometabolic disorders [14]. The type and amount of carbohydrates consumed contribute to the postprandial blood glucose and triglyceride levels, which are associated with oxidative stress and inflammation. Low-GI foods and low-GL diets do not promote a proinflammatory state, whereas high-GI foods and high-GI diets have been shown to induce postprandial hyperglycemia and hypertriglyceridemia, which can potentiate inflammation and oxidative stress [14]. Both the Mediterranean and

Dietary Approaches to Stop Hypertension (DASH) diets incorporate plenty of fresh fruits, vegetables, whole grains, and cardiac healthy fats, many of which are rich in antioxidants that limit the production of damaging free radicals, thereby reducing inflammation and oxidative stress.

Cancer risk

Various studies have implicated high-GI and high-GL diets to be associated with an increased risk for certain types of malignancies. The consumption of a high-GI, high-GL diet leads to chronically elevated serum glucose levels, thereby promoting a chronic state of hyperinsulinemia. This chronic state can lead to insulin resistance associated with the development of NIDDM. At the same time, insulin stimulates the production of the hormone insulin-like growth factor-1, which inhibits cell apoptosis and promotes unregulated cell proliferation, leading to malignant transformation [15, 16]. According to a recent updated metaanalysis published in 2019 by an Italian group, the glycemic index, glycemic load, and cancer risk were rigorously studied and analyzed, demonstrating unfavorable effects of high-GI diets on colorectal, endometrial, bladder, and renal cancers [17].

References

[1] Brand-Miller JC, Holt SH, Pawlak DB, McMillan J. Glycemic index and obesity. Am J Clin Nutr 2002;76:281S–5S.

[2] Boham E, Stone PM, DeBusk R. Obesity. In: Textbook of family medicine. Elsevier; 2016. p. 867–890.e4. Chapter 36.

[3] Jenkins DJA, Wolever TMS, Taylor RH, Barker H, et al. Glycemic index of foods: a physiological basis for carbohydrate exchange. Am J Clin Nutr March 1981;34:362–6.

[4] Brouns F, Bjorck I, Frayn KN, Gibbs AL, et al. Glycaemic index methodology. Nutr Res Rev 2005;18:145–71.

[5] Bjorck I, Granfeldt Y, Liljeberg H, Tovar J, Asp NG. Food properties affecting the digestion and absorption of carbohydrates. Am J Clin Nutr 1994;59:699S–705S.

[6] Rakel D, Onna Lo YM. Glycemic index and glycemic load. In: Integrative medicine. Elsevier; 2018. p. 863–868.e1. Chapter 87.

[7] FAO/WHO Expert Consultation. Carbohydrates in human nutrition: report of a joint FAO/WHO Expert Consultation, Rome, 14–18 April, 1997. Rome: Food and Agriculture Organization; 1998.

[8] Salmeron J, Manson JE, Stampfer MJ, et al. Dietary fiber, glycemic load, and risk of non-insulin-dependent diabetes mellitus in women. JAMA 1997;277:472–7.

[9] Foster-Powell K, Holt SH, Brand-Miller JC. International table of glycemic index and glycemic load values: 2002. Am J Clin Nutr 2002;76:5–56.

[10] Ludwig DS, Majzoub JA, Al-Zahrani A, Dallal GE, et al. High glycemic index foods, overeating, and obesity. Pediatrics 1999;103:863–868.e1.

[11] Maki KC, Rains TM, Kaden VN, Raneri KR, Davidson MH. Effects of a reduced-glycemic-load diet on body weight, body composition, and cardiovascular disease risk markers in overweight and obese adults. Am J Clin Nutr 2007;85:724–34.

[12] Halton TL, Willett WC, Liu S, Manson JE, et al. Low-carbohydrate-diet score and the risk of coronary heart disease in women. N Engl J Med 2006;355:1991–2002.

[13] Liu S, Willett WC, Stampfer MJ, Hu FB, et al. A prospective study of dietary glycemic load, carbohydrate intake, and risk of coronary heart disease in US women. Am J Clin Nutr 2000;71:1455–61.

[14] Egger G, Dixon J. Should obesity be the main game? Or do we need an environmental make-over to combat the inflammatory and chronic disease epidemics? Obes Rev 2009;10:237–49.

[15] Kaaks R, Lukanova A. Energy balance and cancer: the role of insulin and insulin-like growth factor-I. Proc Nutr Soc 2001;60:91–106.

[16] Renehan AG, Zwahlen M, Minder C, et al. Insulin-like growth factor (IGF)-I, IGF binding protein-3, and cancer risk: systematic review and meta-regression analysis. Lancet 2004;363:1346–53.

[17] Turati F, Galeone C, Augustin LS, Vecchia CL. Glycemic index, glycemic load and cancer risk: an updated meta-analysis. Nutrients 2019;11:2342.

Chapter 15

Predictors of obesity

David Kim, M.D.
Department of Surgery, Rhode Island Hospital, Alpert Medical School of Brown University, Providence, RI, United States

Introduction

According to the Centers for Disease Control and Prevention (CDC), obesity in adults is defined as a body mass index (BMI), calculated by weight in kilograms divided by height in meters squared, of ≥ 30 [1]. Obesity in children and adolescents is defined more quantitatively as a BMI at or above the 95th percentile of the CDC sex-specific BMI-for-age growth charts [1].

In the United States, the prevalence of obesity among both adults and children has increased considerably, particularly over the last two decades. Among adults, the prevalence of obesity has increased from 30.5% to 42.4% while the prevalence of those who are severely obese has nearly doubled [1].

Additionally, it is not surprising that obesity has become the most common nutritional disease of children and adolescents in the United States [2]. For children and adolescents aged 2–19 years, the prevalence of obesity was 18.5% with the highest prevalence among adolescents aged 12–19 years at 20.6% [1].

Indeed, obesity affects >13 million US children and is associated with the development of well-documented adverse health consequences into adulthood, including diabetes mellitus and coronary heart disease. Moreover, children who are obese are more likely to carry this extra weight into adulthood, which considerably impacts their overall health and well-being [3].

Childhood and adolescent obesity

Given the detrimental health consequences afflicting those individuals who are severely obese, there has been significant interest in identifying predictors of adult obesity with a focus on prevention and early timing of intervention. A study published in JAMA by Gordon-Larsen et al. at the University of North Carolina (UNC) titled "Association of Adolescent Obesity with Risk of Severe Obesity in Adulthood" aimed to determine the incidence and risk of severe obesity in adulthood by adolescent weight status [4].

Obesity. https://doi.org/10.1016/B978-0-12-818839-2.00015-6

Using the National Longitudinal Study of Adolescent to Adult Health (Add Health) consisting of a cohort of >20,000 adolescents aged 11–20 years in the United States, the group at UNC incorporated 8834 individuals who met their inclusion criteria in their final analytic sample and found that over a 13-year period during the transition from adolescence to adulthood, there were 703 incident cases of severe obesity or an incidence rate of 7.9%. Of those incident cases, certain characteristics such as age, ethnic minorities, and higher adolescent BMI were identified as predictors of obesity [4]. This study illustrated that obesity in adolescence was strongly associated with an increased incidence of severe obesity in adulthood [4].

In a 2010 study published in the *New England Journal of Medicine*, Ward and his colleagues at Harvard examined growth trajectories of childhood obesity into adulthood and generated prediction models by pooling height and weight data from five national longitudinal studies from >40,000 children and adults. Utilizing their rigorous simulation models, the study suggested that the development of obesity in childhood predicted obesity in adulthood [5]. In fact, children who were severely obese were at the highest risk of being obese as adults [5].

From the two representative studies regarding obesity in children and adolescents, the findings underline the importance of timing as well as the value of implementing interventions prior to adulthood to counter weight gain and obesity in an effort to prevent the long-term health effects of obesity in adulthood.

Parental obesity

Understanding that the most meaningful impact on the obesity pandemic likely begins with early interventions specifically targeting children who are obese and severely obese, the contribution of parental obesity or parental BMI as a predictor of future obesity in adulthood has also been studied. In a 1997 retrospective cohort study published in the *New England Journal of Medicine*, Whitaker et al. from the Department of Pediatrics at the University of Cincinnati determined the probability of obesity in adulthood as it relates to the presence or absence of obesity in childhood as well as the presence or absence of parental obesity [6]. In the study, obesity in children was separated into obese children whose BMI was at or above the 85th percentile for age and sex and very obese children whose BMI was at or above the 95th percentile while adult or parental obesity was defined as an average BMI of 27.8 or greater for men and 27.3 or greater for women [6].

Similar to the results presented in the aforementioned section on childhood and adolescent obesity, the researchers found that the risk of obesity in adulthood increased with the age of the obese child, and this risk was higher in children who were very obese [4–6]. In this study, the risk of adult obesity was significantly higher if either parent was obese, and the effect of parental obesity was greatest among children under the age of 10 [6]. Additionally, the subset of children whose BMI was greater than the 95th percentile with one or both parents being obese had the highest risk of adult obesity, demonstrating the contribution of both childhood and parental obesity to the risk of obesity in adulthood [6].

Socioeconomic status

Although childhood and adolescent obesity as well as parental obesity are among the most significant predictors of adult obesity, socioeconomic status has been associated with one's risk for developing obesity [7]. A Finland study published in 2001 by Laitinen et al. illustrated an inverse relationship between obesity and socioeconomic status, that is, a lower social class of a child's family had a higher risk of being obese in adulthood [7]. In addition, using data from a northern Finland birth cohort for 1966, the group identified a high maternal BMI, a high BMI in childhood, and an earlier age of menarche as other predictors of obesity [7].

Home environment

Prior studies have established that the home environment contributes to the risk of childhood obesity. In their 1994 study published in *Lancet*, Lissau-Lund and Sorensen demonstrated that parental neglect during childhood conferred an increased risk of obesity in young adulthood; in fact, this risk was nine times higher in children who were neglected [8].

Strauss and Knight at the University of Medicine and Dentistry of New Jersey sought to better understand the contribution of home environment to childhood obesity [9]. In a prospective cohort study of children enrolled in the National Longitudinal Survey of Youth, Strauss and Knight documented that children with obese mothers, lower socioeconomic factors, and lower cognitive stimulation were all factors that considerably increased their risk of developing obesity, emphasizing the critical role of the home environment in the development of childhood obesity [9].

Physical activity

The development of obesity is multifactorial and complex, and physical activity is certainly a contributing factor. Obesity results from an imbalance where energy intake, typically in the form of calories, exceeds energy expenditure, of which physical activity is a part, among other factors. Salbe and colleagues at the National Institutes of Health revealed that obesity is associated with sedentary lifestyle practices among children, such as decreased participation in sports and increased television viewing [10]. The group reinforced that promoting increased physical activity in children might help attenuate their risk for developing obesity [10].

Dietary factors

Dietary factors that contribute to energy intake can affect the aforementioned energy imbalance that defines obesity. A Spanish study conducted by Rocandio et al. in 2001 implemented a cross-sectional design of 32 school children and recorded dietary intake for a week, defining overweight children with weight-for-height greater than the 90th percentile [11]. Interestingly, in this study, overweight children that were studied did not consume more calories than children who were not overweight, suggesting that the positive energy imbalance causing weight gain may be due to low energy output [11].

Although there has been considerable interest and many studies with the goal of identifying predictors of obesity, it is difficult to discern the relative contribution of each of these predictors given the complex interplay of genetic, environmental, and psychosocial factors to the development of obesity.

References

1. Centers for Disease Control and Prevention. Overweight and obesity, Centers for Disease Control and Prevention; 2020. Retrieved from, http://www.cdc.gov/obesity/index.html.
2. Dietz WH. Health consequences of obesity in youth: childhood predictors of adult disease. Pediatrics 1998;101(3 Pt 2):518–25.
3. Gordon-Larsen P, The NS, Adair LS. Longitudinal trends in obesity in the United States from adolescence to the third decade of life. Obesity 2010;18(9):1801–4.
4. The NS, Suchindran C, North KE, Popkin BM, Gordon-Larsen P. Association of adolescent obesity with risk of severe obesity in adulthood. JAMA 2010 Nov;304(18):2042–7.
5. Ward ZJ, Long MW, Resch SC, Giles CM, et al. Simulation of growth trajectories of childhood obesity into adulthood. N Engl J Med 2017;377:2145–53.
6. Whitaker RC, Wright JA, Pepe MS, et al. Predicting obesity in young adulthood from childhood and parental obesity. N Engl J Med 1997;337:869–73.
7. Laitinen J, Power C, Jarvelin MR. Family social class, maternal body mass index, childhood body mass index, and age at menarche as predictors of adult obesity. Am J Clin Nutr 2001;74:287–94.
8. Lissau-Lund I, TIA S. Parental neglect during childhood and increased risk of obesity in young adulthood. Lancet 1994;343:324–7.
9. Strauss RS, Knight J. Influence of the home environment on the development of obesity in children. Pediatrics 1999;103:e85.
10. Salbe AD, Weyer C, Harper I, Lindsay RS, Ravussin E, Tataranni PA. Assessing risk factors for obesity between childhood and adolescence: II. Energy metabolism and physical activity. Pediatrics 2002;110:307–14.
11. Rocandio AM, Ansotegui L, Arroyo M. Comparison of dietary intake among overweight and nonoverweight school children. Int J Obes Relat Metab Disord 2001;25:1651–5.

Further reading

Boham E, Stone PM, DeBusk R. Obesity. In: Textbook of family medicine. Elsevier; 2016. p. 867–890.e4 [Chapter 36].

Index

Note: Page numbers followed by *f* indicate figures and *t* indicate tables.

MIX
Papier | Fördert
gute Waldnutzung
FSC® C083411

Kolibri 360 GmbH
Ferdinand-Jühlke-Straße 7
99095 Erfurt, Deutschland
produktsicherheit@kolibri360.de